Meeting
the
Realities in
Clinical Teaching

*Ernestine Wiedenbach, R.N., M.A., C.N.M.
Associate Professor Emeritus
of Maternal and Newborn Health Nursing,
Yale University*

MEETING THE REALITIES IN CLINICAL TEACHING

Ernestine Wiedenbach

Springer Publishing Company, Inc., New York

Copyright, © 1969
SPRINGER PUBLISHING COMPANY, INC.
200 Park Avenue South, New York, N. Y. 10003

All rights reserved

Library of Congress Catalog Card Number: 75-78917

Printed in U. S. A.

Preface

Meeting the Realities in Clinical Teaching is presented as a companion to *Clinical Nursing: A Helping Art,* published in 1964. At the time the earlier book was written, the concept of a prescriptive theory as a guide to practice had not, in its entirety, become a conscious part of my nursing practice or my teaching. However, some of its components—particularly purpose, prescription in the form of deliberative action, and aspects of the realities—are discernible in the earlier book, and may be recognized as factors that exerted a strong influence on the nurse's actions in the various situations described. In the present book, the components of such a theory are individually distinguished and their relationship to practice is made explicit. Writing it has given me clarity about the importance of each component to clinical teaching and to the outcome the instructor hopes to effect through what she does.

I was introduced to the significance of a prescriptive theory in a practice discipline by Drs. William J. Dickoff and Patricia A. James, philosophers at Yale University, whom I happily regard as my good friends. To them I express my deep appreciation for the generous way in which they shared with me their concepts of the several levels of theory and the importance of each to practice and research. Applying some of those concepts to the practice of clinical teaching, as I have tried to do in this book, has been a challenging and revealing experience. In spite of over 20 years of participation in clinical teaching programs, I think I would not have undertaken this task at this time had Dorothy M. Smith, Dean of the College of Nursing at the University of Florida, not given me the opportunity, in the summer of 1968, to teach in a special masters program at the College. This enabled me to make direct application of some of the concepts and to check their validity. I am grateful also to Jennet Wilson, chairman of the maternal-infant nursing section, who gave constant support to my efforts throughout our close association that summer.

When developed according to a prescriptive theory, a clinical teaching program gains, I have discovered, substance, trenchancy, and stature. It enables students not only to gain knowledge and skills, but also to apply them in practice and to obtain desired results. The purpose, goal, and objectives of the program are given practical meaning, and such commitments as planning, orienting, and evaluating, which often are taken for granted, are recognized as vital to its effectiveness. A program thus developed cannot be lightly undertaken. Its implementation calls for wisdom, perspicacity, and thoughtful review and assessment of actions.

For the content of this book, I have drawn heavily on my experiences in clinical teaching at the Yale University School of Nursing and at the College of Nursing, University of Florida. I am deeply indebted to the students whom I was privileged to teach for their responsiveness and their ideals. The inspiration to write this book, however, was generated by my association with young instructors in university schools of nursing across this continent, particularly (in addition to those at Yale and at the University of Florida) those at California State University in Los Angeles, Capital University in Columbus, Ohio, University of Kansas, Ohio State University, University of Southern Mississippi in Hattiesburg, University of Utah, University of Western Ontario, and Wisconsin State University in Eau Claire. These instructors represent many fields of nursing, including maternal and infant health, medical, surgical, psychiatric, and public health. It was heartening to note that they readily saw how the concepts that are expounded here had relevance for their areas of special interest, even though many

PREFACE

of the examples I presented to them were drawn, as are those in this book, from my special field—maternal and newborn health nursing. I sincerely appreciate the opportunities I had to exchange ideas with these young faculty members, to learn of their aspirations and frustrations, and to witness their earnest desire to enable their students to become competent practitioners of nursing.

Credit for the preparation of the illustrative charts in this book goes to Caroline E. Falls, whose friendship I have valued for many years. I am deeply grateful for her untiring effort to capture the meaning of concepts and incorporate it in her drawings, for her unfailing encouragement during the preparation of the manuscript, and for her many helpful and practical suggestions for strengthening its content.

I also wish to express appreciation to Mrs. Helen Behnke who edited the manuscript with expertise and sensitivity.

ERNESTINE WIEDENBACH

Woodbury, Connecticut
March, 1969

Contents

I INTRODUCTION	1
II CENTRAL PURPOSE IN CLINICAL TEACHING	6
III PRESCRIPTION FOR CLINICAL TEACHING	11
IV THE REALITIES IN CLINICAL TEACHING	18
The Agent: The Clinical Instructor	21
Reconciliation of the instructor's assumptions	22
Specification of the instructor's objectives	25
Formulation of plans	28
. *What needs to be planned?*	28
What specific plans need to be made?	29
. . *Course of study*	29
Student experience	31
Preparation of instructor	34
Students' preparation for clinical experience	35
. . . *Individual conferences*	36
Group conferences	36
Rehearsal for practice	36
A tour	37
Informative written material	37
. . *Students' time schedule*	39
Evaluation of students' participation	44
. . . *Provision for self-disclosure*	45
Provision for first-hand knowledge	45
Specification of desirable attributes	45
Construction of system of symbols	47
Assignment of numerical value	48
Construction of a score form	49
Summarization of scores	51
Provision for discussion of scores	52
. . *Participation of nursing staff*	52
Teaching staff's responsibilities	54

. How can implementation be assured? 55
Implementation of plans 57
Toward self realization and improvement of practice 60
. Further study 61
Purposeful practice of nursing 62
Nursing research 63
Relevant writing for publication 64
The Recipient: The Student 66
Ten assumptions 71
The Framework 83
The Goal 95
The Means 102
Classes and conferences 103
Clinical experience 106
. Preparatory conferences 107
. . A tour of the area 107
Introduction to personnel 108
Rounds 108
Demonstrations 109
Rehearsal for practice 110
. Briefing conferences 114
Tutorial practice 115
. . Asking the student to confer 116
Going to the area where student is 117
Making opportunistic contact 119
. Post-experience conferences 120
Assignments 121
. Reconstruction of nursing incidents 123
Special projects 135
Summaries of thinking 138
Tests and evaluations 142
Teaching and learning aids 152

V. SUMMARY 157

REFERENCES 161

INDEX 163

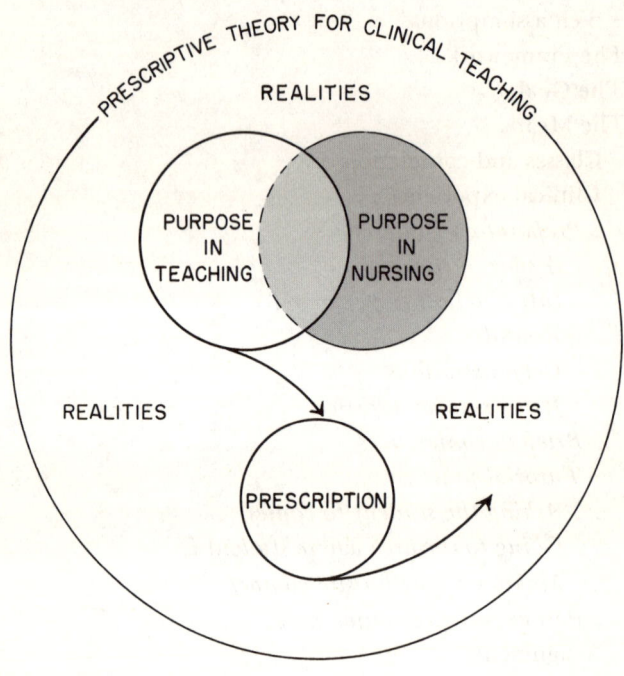

1

Introduction

Clinical teaching, the art of enabling a student to develop her potential for safe, effective, competent functioning within the realities of the immediate clinical situation, may be thought of as an extension of academic teaching. Whereas academic teaching enables the student to assimilate, understand, excerpt and store essentials of subject matter as resources for future enjoyment, application or use, clinical teaching enables the student to translate learned subject matter into practical knowledge and to apply it meaningfully within the realities of the clinical situation.

Teaching may be described as action designed to enable an individual to learn; and learning as the process of assimilating knowledge or developing skills for either academic or practical use.

In general, the aim of academic teaching may be said to be achieved when the student gives evidence, through a variety of verbal or graphic testing devices, that she has assimilated and understands essentials of subject matter taught. The aim of clinical teaching, on the other hand, is achieved when the student gives evidence that she understands the subject matter taught by competently applying appropriate portions of it within the realities of a clinical situation and thereby effecting desired results. Thus, clinical teaching imposes a twofold responsibility on the instructor: 1) competence in the discipline of teaching; and 2) competence in the clinical discipline taught.

Nursing, a clinical discipline, is—like teaching—a practice discipline. This means that both nursing and teaching represent activities that are goal-directed, i.e., designed to produce explicit results of a desired kind within the realities of specified existing and future situations.

Underlying a practice discipline that is professional in character* is a prescriptive theory also known as a situation-producing theory. Theory has been described as a system of conceptualizations invented to some purpose; while a situation-producing theory (prescriptive theory) may be described as one which conceptualizes both a desired situation and the prescription by which it is to be brought about. Thus, a prescriptive theory directs action toward an explicit goal.

In relation to a practice discipline such as nursing, medicine or teaching, a prescriptive theory may be said to specify action the practitioner must take in order to bring about a result deemed desirable in the context of the discipline. This presumes that in articulating a prescriptive theory for a practice discipline, three distinct factors must be taken into account.

1. The central purpose which the practitioner recognizes as essential to the particular discipline.
2. The prescription for fulfillment of the central purpose.
3. The realities in the immediate situation that influence fulfillment of the central purpose.

1. *Central purpose* represents the practitioner's concept of the mission to be accomplished through his implementation of the concepts basic to the discipline. By suggesting both the direction and nature of the action he will take, it becomes his professional commitment. Thus it reflects both his view of the overall goal of the discipline and his own beliefs and values.

---

* "A true professional—as opposed to a mere visionary—shapes reality according to an articulate purpose and in the light of means conceptualized in relation not only to purpose but also in relation to existent reality." James Dickoff and Patricia James, "A Theory of Theories: A Position Paper." In Symposium on Theory Development in Nursing. *Nurs. Research* 17:3, May-June, 1968, p. 199.

It is of great importance for the clinical instructor to articulate her purpose in teaching explicitly, for only then can it be apprehended and its validity ascertained. By articulating it she also converts it into a practical tool that she can use as a standard by which to measure the effectiveness of her acts and as a guide in her efforts to enhance her consistency and reliability in her practice. Articulation of purpose gives it a personal quality and, consequently, it is designated as purpose *in* (rather than *of*) clinical teaching. This personal connotation also implies that the practitioner can subject her purpose to examination and refinement as she gains new insights from thoughtfully reviewed experiences.

2. *Prescription* is a directive to activity. For a practice discipline, it may indicate the broad general actions appropriate to implementation of the basic concepts of the discipline, and also suggest the kind of behavior needed to carry out these actions in accordance with the central purpose.

Action may be voluntary or involuntary. As conceived here, voluntary action is an intended response to a stimulus originating within the realities of the immediate situation, while involuntary action is an unintended response.

As part of a situation-producing theory, prescription is a directive to at least three kinds of voluntary action:

    a. Mutually understood and agreed-upon
    b. Recipient-directed
    c. Practitioner-directed

Mutually understood and agreed-upon implies that the practitioner has obtained evidence that the recipient understands the implications of the intended action and is psychologically, physically and/or physiologically receptive to it.

Recipient-directed implies that the recipient of the action essentially directs the way in which it is to be carried out.

Practitioner-directed implies that the practitioner carries out the action according to his notion of its appropriateness, value or importance.

The three kinds of voluntary action may be diagrammed as shown at the top of the next page.

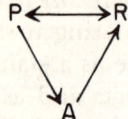 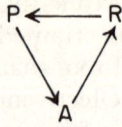 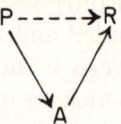

Mutually understood and agreed-upon action | Recipient-directed action | Practitioner-directed action

(P = practitioner; R = recipient; A = action)

In a practice discipline such as nursing, the close relationship that exists between central purpose and prescription suggests that both are influenced by beliefs that are the basis of the practitioner's working philosophy. When such a philosophy is made explicit, it gives substance to her commitment, guides her thinking about the nature of her actions, and influences her resultant decisions.

3. The *realities* of the immediate situation constitute the matrix within which action occurs. They are essentially five in number and may be designated as:

1. *The agent* who is the practitioner (or his delegate) and who supplies the propelling force for any action that may be taken.
2. *The recipient* who receives the agent's action or in whose behalf the action is taken.
3. *The framework* that comprises all the extraneous factors and facilities in the situation that affect the practitioner's ability to obtain the kind of results he wants to obtain through what he does within the context of his discipline.
4. *The goal* that represents the end to be attained through the activity the agent plans or undertakes in behalf of the recipient.
5. *The means* that comprise the activities and devices through which the practitioner is enabled to attain his goal.

The realities give uniqueness to every situation encountered. To a large degree, the success of professional practice hinges on them, for unless they are recognized in prescription and effectively dealt with, they may present insuperable obstacles to achievement of the goal and to the fulfillment of the practitioner's central purpose in engaging in the discipline.

Central purpose, prescription and realities, thus, are inextricably tied up with one another. Together, they constitute the substance of any prescriptive theory which, when articulated, serves as the guiding light of professional practice.

Central Purpose in Clinical Teaching

Central purpose in clinical teaching,* when formulated and made explicit by the instructor, becomes a point of reference that gives direction to her teaching and helps her to maintain her focus. When the instructor is a nurse—and she almost always is—her central purpose in clinical teaching becomes teamed with her central purpose in nursing but, except in emergencies, is maintained in a dominant role. This means that the instructor is responsible for enabling the student to experience and cope with situations that are conducive to her growth and development as a practitioner of nursing while, at the same time, the instructor is accountable both for what the student does in the clinical situation and for the results the student gets from her nursing action. For the instructor to recognize the relationship between her two purposes, and to function effectively in their fulfillment, calls for clarity about each of them and for judgment of high order in deciding what actions are to be taken to fulfill them.

The danger always exists that the instructor may become caught on the horns of a dilemma because of a conflict of interests. Although, by virtue of her instructor's role, the focus of her attention is the student, her interest tends to be twofold: teaching the student and caring for the patient. Indeed, the in-

---

* In the following chapters, the term *clinical teaching* refers to clinical teaching in the field of nursing unless otherwise specified.

CENTRAL PURPOSE 7

structor may feel more confident, competent and comfortable in giving patient care than she does in teaching the student, particularly if she is new to the area of clinical teaching.

The following incidents illustrate the kinds of conflict situations that may present such a dilemma to the clinical instructor at almost any time in the course of a day's teaching activities in the clinical area.

1. The clinical instructor enters a patient's room just as a student is about to catheterize the patient. As she nears the bed, she observes the patient's anxious expression and senses the tension of the student who, she notes, with consternation, is awkwardly trying to keep the patient's labia separated with one hand while with the other she is shakingly holding the catheter and attempting to insert it into a fold of tissue immediately below the urinary meatus which is barely discernible.

2. A student who is caring for a cardiac patient in a 4-bed room is unable to count the patient's pulse and has asked the clinical instructor's help. Just as the instructor is about to enter the screened-off area where the student and the patient are, she hears a patient in one of the other beds call out anxiously, "Nurse, please give me a bedpan. I can't wait."

3. A clinical instructor is accompanying a student who, for the first time, is about to give an enema to a mother in labor. The mother recognizes the instructor as they approach the bed and, with a note of relief exclaims, "Oh, Miss Jones, I'm so glad you are still here. I've been dreading this enema because of my hemorrhoids, remember?" Then, glancing at the student and back to the instructor, the mother added, "You'll give it to me again this time, won't you? Please!"

4. Every bed in the surgical unit is filled and only three or four patients are up and around. The few nurses on the understaffed unit are valiantly trying to keep up with the patients' various needs. Aides help out wherever they

can, but more staff nurses are needed. The students assigned to the unit are involved in caring for their patients and seem to be managing well. The clinical instructor has made the rounds of her students and, for the time being, feels herself to be at loose ends. She has spotted an elderly patient who looks as though he feels miserable. She would like to do something to relieve his discomfort, but wonders if she should allow herself to become involved in his care.

The action the clinical instructor might take in any of these situations will be based on the judgment that she makes at the moment of taking it. Her judgment, however, may be swayed by such feelings as distress, compassion or concern for the patient. Should she let her feelings mainly guide her action, she runs the risk of either failing the student or of alienating the patient. Should she base her action solely on her purpose in nursing and take over the care of the patient, she would be disregarding the needs of the student. Should she respond solely on the basis of her purpose in clinical teaching, she might disregard the needs of the patient and, as pointed out in some of the instances cited, this could irritate the patient and aggravate his condition. In addition, it might rouse feelings of distress and distrust in the student because the patient's need had been ignored. If, however, the clinical instructor is clear about her purpose in clinical teaching and its relationship to her purpose in nursing, she will be likely to decide on an action that will uphold her commitment to her student and, at the same time, fulfill her responsibility to the patient.

A statement of purpose in nursing that the author has formulated and which a number of practitioners of nursing subscribe to and follow is:

> To motivate the individual and/or facilitate her efforts to overcome the obstacles that now—or may later—interfere with her ability to respond capably to the demands made of her by the realities in the health situation of which she is a part.

A corollary for clinical teaching might be:

> To motivate the student and/or facilitate her efforts to overcome the obstacles that now—or may later—interfere with her ability to gain the knowledge, insights and skills she needs to function capably, as a nurse, within the realities of the situation of which she is or may become a part.

This corollary suggests that the clinical instructor's overall goal is the student's capability as a nurse. It also suggests that she will be most likely to attain that goal by facilitating the student's efforts to gain knowledge, skill and insights. Finally, it implies that her beliefs include faith in the student's ability and desire to learn, once interfering obstacles are overcome.

Three basic concepts underlie these statements of purpose and can serve as a frame of reference for the clinical instructor in making choices and decisions. They are:

1. Reverence for the gift of life and for the ability to live and learn.
2. Respect for the dignity, worth, autonomy and individuality of each human being.
3. Resolution to act dynamically in relation to one's beliefs.

Of these concepts, the second probably exerts the greatest influence on the instructor's attitude toward the student. Four basic assumptions that give validity to this concept are:

1. Each human being is endowed with unique potential to develop personal resources that enable him to maintain and sustain himself.
2. Basically, the human being strives toward self-direction and relative independence, and desires to make the best use of his capabilities and potentialities and to fulfill his responsibilities.
3. Self-awareness and self-acceptance are essential to the individual's sense of integrity and self-worth.

4. Whatever the individual does represents his best judgment at the moment of doing it.

Every clinical instructor is urged to think through, enunciate and clarify her central purpose in teaching and the beliefs that underlie it. This will contribute to her confidence and constancy in teaching, for it will demonstrate that she knows what results she wants to obtain through her teaching and her reasons for wanting to obtain them.

III

Prescription for Clinical Teaching

Prescription in clinical teaching parallels prescription in medicine in many ways. In medicine, prescription signifies not only substances that are to be combined to form a particular medication, but also how the medication is to be used in order to effect the changes that the physician hopes to bring about in the patient. Similarly, in clinical teaching, prescription indicates the factors that, when combined, give direction to the instructor's action as well as to the thinking process that, hopefully, will lead to the results desired by the instructor.

Action in any practice discipline is goal-directed. In clinical teaching, the goal toward which action is directed is the development of the student's nursing competence. Nursing competence, however, is something that the student must develop for and within herself. Therefore, the clinical instructor's function is to motivate the student to try to develop the kind of competence the instructor deems desirable, and to be responsive to the instructor's method of teaching.

Professional action—and clinical teaching may be so termed—is based on a thinking process that always precedes the action, whether it be verbal or non-verbal in form. This process entails apprehension of the practitioner's central purposes and their relationship to each other, and of the realities in the situation, as well as any assumption the instructor may have made about the meaning of the student's attitude and/or behavior.

This thinking process derives, generally, from a stimulus originating in the realities in the situation, for example, a question asked by a student; a procedure the instructor observes a student carrying out; or a request that the instructor hears the head nurse make for a student to give a treatment that the instructor knows the student has never given before. This stimulus reaches the instructor through her sensory organs and is passed to the central nervous system where it is interpreted as a sensation. Her awareness of the sensation could result in a reflex action on her part, but it is more likely to be converted into a perception. The perception could give rise to a conditioned type of action, but it is more apt to result in an assumption. The assumption could give rise to impulsive action (emotional response to an unvalidated assumption) that might have unfortunate consequences. If, however, the instructor realizes that the assumption stems from *her* perception of some aspect of the realities, she may avoid this danger by abruptly halting the imaginings, speculations and emotions that precede impulsive action, thus giving herself opportunity to recognize the explosive nature of her feeling-charged thoughts. Such an act of halting may be referred to as the application of a strategy brake.

Sensations, perceptions and assumptions are conscious but involuntary phenomena, and so may be said to occur automatically. Although they come unbidden into the instructor's consciousness, each of them may serve to incite definitive action that, no matter what its form, will have an altering effect on the realities from which the original stimulus derived and on the instructor's immediate intent. The following examples illustrate how definitive actions may be brought about automatically:

> A. *Reflex action resulting from a sensation:* An instructor picks up the removable lid of a sterilizing pan without realizing that the hot plate on which it is sitting has just been turned off. The lid is piping hot, she drops it, it misses the pan and falls to the floor. In this example, the act of letting go of the lid (reflex action) has an altering

effect on the pan and lid relationship (part of the realities) and necessitates a change in plans from whatever the instructor's intent had been when she started to remove the lid from the pan.

B. *Conditioned action resulting from a perception:* An instructor's office has been moved from the third to the ground floor. For years, on arriving at school, she has gone directly to the elevator and taken it to the third floor. On the morning after the move, she enters the building and heads, as usual, for the elevator, steps aboard and punches the third-floor button. She does not realize her mistake until the elevator door opens to let her off. In this illustration, the instructor's adherence to the pattern of taking the elevator (conditioned action) has an altering effect on her (as part of the realities), once she realizes her absent-mindedness; it also alters her original intent to go directly to her new office upon entering the building.

C. *Impulsive action resulting from an unvalidated assumption:* A student is supporting Mrs. Green, a mother who is in early labor. The instructor is about to enter the labor room when the head nurse calls to her, "Do you want your student to observe a section? She'll have to hurry, for they are just about to start one on Mrs. Jones."

The instructor responds, "Oh, yes. Thanks!" She then quickly enters the labor room, beckons the student to her, and tells her to go immediately to the delivery room to observe the section. The student demurs. The instructor says, "Hurry, or you'll miss it. I'll stay with Mrs. Green."

As the student continues to hesitate, the instructor, with mounting annoyance, says sharply, "Go on, I'm telling you. Stop dallying!"

At that, the student bursts into tears and in a barely perceptible voice says, "No, I can't. I'm afraid to see it!"

In this example, the instructor's sharp command (impulsive action), based on the assumption that the student is needlessly delaying or willfully disobeying, has an altering effect on the realities (the student and the situation in which she was functioning) and on the instructor's own intent to stay with Mrs. Green while the student observes the section.

Reflex, conditioned and impulsive actions can be extremely valuable—even lifesaving—at times. They are uncontrolled by reason, however, and useful as they may be at times of emergency, should not be allowed to predominate in the actions taken by the clinical instructor.

Impulsive action on the part of the instructor is a common cause of student distress and instructor frustration. To guard against taking such action, the onrush of feelings that so often complicate assumptions must be brought under control. The instructor can learn to do this by schooling herself to "stop, look and listen," in other words, to apply a strategy brake whenever she becomes aware of such upsurging feelings, or whenever she realizes that she is about to act on an unvalidated assumption. Her emotions may frequently be aroused by assumptions about the perception of a stimulus that she received from the realities in the immediate situation, and her assumptions, unless validated, are unilateral in character. They represent the meaning *she* attaches to her perception on the basis of *her* frame of reference. Application of a strategy brake to rampant feelings provides time for the instructor to examine her assumptions with objectivity in light of her purpose in clinical teaching and the realities in the situation. This, in effect, harnesses her feelings to disciplined thoughts and brings them under conscious control. From such examination, the instructor may gain insight into the character and validity of her assumptions, and then she will be able to come to a deliberate decision about what action to take (see diagram, p. 15).

On the basis of the thinking process just described, the four steps that lead to deliberate action in clinical teaching and to a prescription for clinical teaching are:

PRESCRIPTION

1. An assumption regarding the instructor's perception of the stimulating aspects of the realities in the situation.
2. A strategy brake.
3. An articulated central purpose in clinical teaching.
4. The realities in the situation.

Of these factors, purpose that derives from an explicit philosophy may be said to exert the greatest influence on the specific nature of ensuing deliberate action.

When an instructor consistently displays in her teaching practice one of the three kinds of action described earlier (see pp. 12-24), her actions quite probably reflect her central purpose

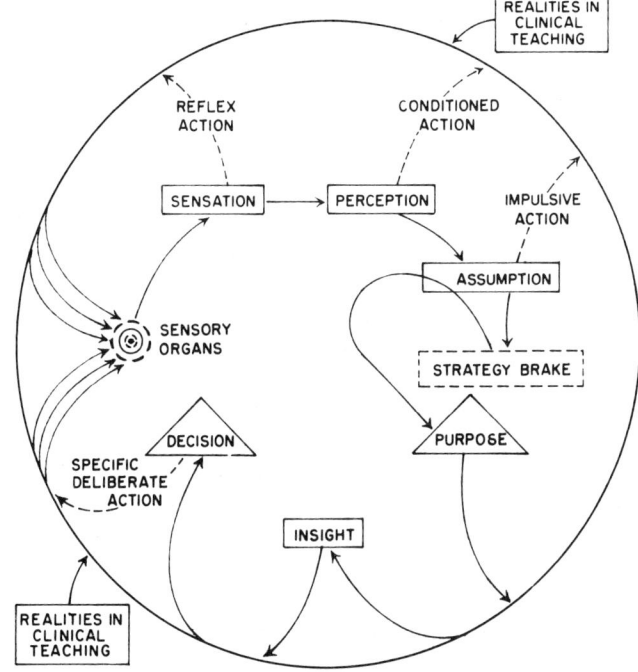

THE GENESIS OF DELIBERATE ACTION

Schematic presentation of how a stimulus emanating from within the realities in the clinical situation is converted into an impulse that can lead to deliberate action. Broken lines represent overt (external, observable) action; solid lines represent covert (internal, not observable) action.

in teaching and the beliefs that underlie it. Mutually understood and agreed-upon action, for example, suggests that the instructor respects the student's dignity, worth, individuality and autonomy. It indicates, too, that she believes that the student must be psychologically receptive to the instructor's teaching if she is to learn from it. For this kind of action, the instructor's central purpose may be said to be: to motivate the student and/or facilitate her efforts to realize her potential for responding capably to the demands made of her by the realities in the learning situation of which she is a part. In all probability, the effect of this kind of action will be positive, and the student will be receptive to the instructor's teaching.

Student-directed action suggests that the instructor respects the student's dignity, worth, individuality and autonomy but that she believes the student knows what she wants to learn and that she will let the instructor know what her learning needs are. It implies that the instructor's central purpose is to support the student in what she assumes is the student's desire—to maintain or attain independence in her clinical practice. The effect this kind of action may have on the student could be positive or it could be negative. The student may be receptive to this way of teaching or she may be frustrated by it.

Instructor-directed action suggests that the instructor may respect the student's dignity, worth and individuality, but not her autonomy. It implies that the instructor believes it is she who knows best what the student is to learn. For this kind of action, the instructor's central purpose would seem to be to tell the student what to do and how to do it. The effect of such action will—in all probability—be negative, for although the student may submit to the instructor's directions, she may also be resentful, even rebellious.

The relationship between the instructor's central purpose, the prescriptive action she takes, and the probable effect of this action on the student may be summarized as shown at the top of the next page.

If the outline shown of the causal relationship between the clinical instructor's central purpose, her action and its effect seems credible, then mutually understood and agreed-upon ac-

PRESCRIPTION

Clinical instructor's central purpose	Clinical instructor's prescriptive action	Probable effect of action on student
To motivate the student and/or facilitate her efforts to realize her potential for responding capably to the demands made of her by the realities of the learning situation of which she is part	Mutually understood and agreed-upon action I ⇄ S ＼ ／ A	Receptive to the instructor's teaching
To support the student in her assumed desire to maintain or attain independence in her practice	Student-directed action I ← S ＼ ／ A	Receptive to instructor's way of teaching, or frustrated by it
To tell the student what she is to do and how she is to do it	Instructor-directed action I - - - → S ＼ ／ A	Submissive and/or resentful, even rebellious

I = Instructor; S = Student; A = Action

tion would seem to be the kind most likely to lead to desired results.

In this chapter, prescription for clinical teaching has been described as a directive for effecting in the student the kind of results desired by the clinical instructor. Of necessity, then, prescription is dependent on the instructor's central purpose in clinical teaching. Once she has formulated it and has accepted it as her commitment, she not only will have established the prescription for her teaching, but she should also be ready to implement it within the realities of the clinical teaching situation.

IV

The Realities in Clinical Teaching

The realities in clinical teaching comprise all of the factors that influence the development and implementation of a clinical teaching program and that affect the instructor's ability to obtain the kind of results she desires from what she does. These factors may be human and non-human; that is, they may be physical, physiological, psychological and/or spiritual. They exist in unpredictable combinations and forms and manifest themselves in an unlimited variety of ways. Regardless of their manifestations, they always are forces that must be recognized and reckoned with, for they exert powerful influences, sometimes obviously, often subtly, on the instructor's ability to carry out her teaching commitment.

The realities inevitably enter into every clinical teaching effort in which the clinical instructor may engage. Each of them can contribute in a vital and significant way to the success, or failure, of her effort. Consequently, it is important for her to recognize each of them, to examine the assumptions she makes about each in light of her central purpose in clinical teaching and, if necessary, bring each into harmony with it. Such reconciliation will go far toward enabling her to cope with the demands in the situation with tolerance, confidence and courage, and with a deepened understanding of her responsibilities and her potential for meeting them.

One of the most influential realities that the instructor has to deal with is the clinical setting where students gain experience in the practice of nursing. Nursing educators often refer to it as a *nursing laboratory*. But many clinical instructors regard such designation as a gross misnomer. To them, the hospital units, the emergency room and the other areas where life dramas are enacted daily, are not related in any way to the scientist's laboratory where action is controlled and carried on according to predetermined specifications. The term "laboratory" could more accurately be used to designate the "nursing arts" classroom where students begin to develop nursing skills under reasonably controlled conditions according to predetermined routines that are usually described in a procedure book. But then, just as the scientist, in order to establish the value of his laboratory findings, applies his findings within the realities of life situations, so the student, in order to establish the meaningfulness of her classroom learning, must apply it within the realities of the clinical situation.

The clinical setting needs to be recognized for what it is: a place in a hospital or health center where both patients and personnel are engaged in restoring health and preserving life; where a variety of actions are engaged in by individuals of varying backgrounds, competencies and purposes; and where the nurse is expected to exercise both judgment and skill in her implementation—within the context of the realities—of services needed for and by the patient.

In clinical teaching, too, the realities are largely responsible for the clinical instructor's need to exercise judgment in the fulfillment of her purpose. They give shape, excitement and uniqueness to every experienced situation and, by their very existence, frequently make it necessary for the instructor to adjust a prescribed course of action in order to get the results she desires.

The realities in clinical teaching may be grouped under five major headings:

1. The agent
2. The recipient
3. The framework
4. The goal
5. The means

Each of these realities is a significant aspect of the total clinical teaching complex, and each calls for thoughtful recognition and consideration by the clinical instructor, not only as she plans her program of clinical teaching but also as she goes about its execution. Although, as aspects of the total clinical teaching complex, the five basic realities are interrelated and interdependent, each may be considered an entity in its own right. Therefore, the remainder of Part III of this book is devoted to descriptions of these realities with respect to their individual characteristics and pertinence for clinical teaching, and the significance that each may hold for the clinical instructor.

● ● ● ● ● ● ● ● ● ● ● ●

The Agent: The Clinical Instructor

The agent in the clinical teaching complex is the clinical instructor and, as such, she supplies the propelling force for the overt actions that determine the effectiveness of her teaching. Results of her teaching are obtained through what she does and how she does it. This implies that she is responsible for clarifying her central purpose in clinical teaching and her prescription for fulfilling it, and also for recognizing the commitments that are hers by virtue of her resolve to fulfill her purpose and implement her prescription. Commitments may be personal in nature and have no direct relevance to clinical teaching, for example, those that derive from prejudice or promises. Others, however, are general in character and are directly relevant to her teaching, for example, those that derive from her respect for her central purpose and her prescription. Five of these general commitments that stand out because they influence the quality of the instructor's teaching in the clinical area are her commitment to:

1. Reconcile her assumptions about the realities in the clinical situation with her central purpose in clinical teaching.
2. Specify her objectives for students' learning in terms of behavioral outcomes that are realistically attainable.
3. Formulate plans for student learning within the realities of the school and clinical setting.
4. Implement the plans.
5. Engage in related activities that contribute to her self-realization and to improvement of nursing practice.

Each of these commitments presumes that the instructor has at least three following qualifications:

1. Knowledgeableness and perceptiveness in her area of special interest with respect to substantive and theoretic content as well as to existing and available general resources and facilities.
2. Adaptability and competence not only in making practical application of her knowledge herself, but also in enabling the student to acquire knowledge and apply it in the clinical situation.
3. Familiarity with the special resources in the school, hospital and community upon which she may draw in developing her program.

The five commitments bear elaboration, for unless their meaning is understood, their significance may not be recognized; therefore, the next several paragraphs will present material that was used in developing an actual clinical teaching program in nursing. Although it proved useful in one program, it in no sense represents an accepted standard. It is meant to be suggestive only. Hopefully, it will stimulate the instructor to think through the many facets of her role in clinical teaching and, when appropriate, to commit her thoughts to paper. In that way she will be able to examine, re-examine and revise them as new insights come to her with time, experience and thought.

Commitment No. 1.
Reconciliation of the instructor's assumptions about the realities with her central purpose in clinical teaching

The instructor's perception of the realities and her resultant assumptions about them, may constitute the key to her effectiveness in functioning within them. To turn the key and unlock the door, however, she needs to reconcile her assumptions with her central purpose in clinical teaching. Only after she has done this will her awareness of how she views the individual realities in a situation, and her interpretation of their meaning, give true direction to what she must do. Every situation in which the instructor finds herself makes some sort of demands of her. These may come from within herself, as when, sitting at a desk in the unit's office, she thinks she should go to room 258 to see how her student is getting along. Or, they may come directly from a student, a patient, the head nurse, ward maid or doctor. They may even come from such inanimate sources as a mineral oil bottle lying smashed at her feet, or a directive in the form of a memo from someone in the "front office." How she views her role in relation to the situation determines her intent to deal with it, and how she views her ability to deal with the demands she senses, determines the action she may take. This view of her role and of herself is important. It stems from the philosophy underlying her central purpose in clinical teaching and from her clarity about both her philosophy and her purpose. Since philosophy may be defined as an integrated and consistent personal attitude toward life and reality, her view of her role and of herself influences not only how she regards each of the other factors within the realities of the immediate situation, but also how she responds to the demands made of her and the results she obtains from her responsive acts.

For example, if the clinical instructor realizes that this role imposes on her the responsibility to be readily available and supportive to the student in her effort to learn from her clinical experience, and if the instructor assumes further that she is potentially able to support the student in her learning effort in a way that will be accepted, then the instructor will not only go to room 258 where the student is, but she will go with confidence in her ability to give the student any help that she may need. Concomitantly, and hopefully with consciousness, her confidence in her own potential to help will cause the instructor to view the student as potentially able to respond positively to the instructor's presence and support, and her intent will undoubtedly be to enable the student to benefit from her teaching. Then, the fact that this instructor has decided to go to the student suggests that she views the nursing staff and others in the area as potentially supportive and feels reasonably assured that it is permissible and possible, so far as policy and environment are concerned, for her to go to room 258. Finally, because

DETERMINANTS OF THE CLINICAL

If the clinical instructor assumes that: As agent she is:	The recipient (student) as:	The clinical framework as:
Potentially competent, and committed to motivating the student and/or facilitating her effort to realize her potential for responding capably to the demands made of her by the realities in the learning situation	Potentially capable	Potentially supportive
Essentially competent, and committed to encouraging the student to be independent in her response to demands made of her by the realities in the learning situation	Essentially capable	Pliable
Competent, and committed to teaching the student to respond with compliance to the demands made of her by the realities in the learning situation	Currently incapable	Essentially supportive

of her commitment and her assumption about her competence, when the instructor reaches the room, she will, in all probability, seek evidence that the student is receptive to her presence and, upon obtaining it, will support the student's learning effort according to the student's indication of need for such support and her receptivity to it.

The causal relationship that exists between the clinical instructor's perception and resultant assumptions about the realities in the situation of which she is a part, and the outcome of

REALITIES

INSTRUCTOR'S COURSE OF ACTION

instructor will recognize:

Her goal as:	The means as:	The probable outcome of the instructor's action with respect to the student will be:
The student's capability	Teaching expedients carried out through mutually understood and agreed-upon action: 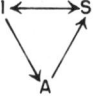	Receptivity toward her (the instructor's) teaching
The student's independence	Teaching expedients carried out through student-directed action: 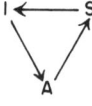	a. Receptivity toward her (the instructor's) teaching b. Frustration
The student's compliance	Teaching expedients carried out through instructor-directed action: 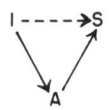	a. Compliance with her (the instructor's) instruction b. Resentfulness c. Rebellion

I = Instructor;
S = Student; A = Action

action she takes as a result of them, is implied in the foregoing example, but may more readily be discerned in the above chart.

Commitment No. 2.
Specification of the instructor's objectives for student learning

Objectives for student learning represent the various kinds of skills and capabilities the instructor thinks are essential for the student to acquire in order to function competently within the realities in the clinical situation. They are hoped-for outcomes and as such they may serve as a blueprint for the instructor when setting up her course by suggesting the kinds of learning experiences to seek for her students. They may also serve the student by letting her know what the instructor's expectations for her learning are.

To be meaningful, objectives need to be realistically attainable, and the degree of their attainment needs to be measurable. This becomes possible when objectives are expressed in terms of behavioral competencies. Competence encompasses both skill, which is defined as deft, dexterous action, and capability—defined as adroit, purposeful handling of situations. It also implies a thinking process that is based on knowledge and leads to understanding, thus causing action that is taken to be appropriate, goal-directed, timely, adequate and effective. Competence, however, is a concept. It is not a substantive, tangible entity and therefore is not, of itself, subject to measurement. Nevertheless, it may be measured, partly by the manner in which action is carried out and especially by the results obtained from the action. For example, a student who rubs the back of a restless patient to soothe him, will be considered competent in the execution of that procedure if, as she gently rubs his back, he comments about how good it feels and subsequently falls asleep. She will be considered less than competent, however, if, as she vigorously rubs his back, he winces, tenses, draws away from her and asks her to stop.

The instructor's objectives for student learning then, may be termed desirable behavioral competencies that, hopefully, the student will acquire through her clinical nursing experience. In formulating them, the instructor needs to keep in mind her central purposes in clinical teaching and in nursing. These represent the overall goals toward which she is constantly striving and, consequently, consistency between them and her objectives for her students' learning is essential.

The following list of objectives is presented in the hope that it will stimulate clinical instructors to examine their own objectives in order to assess their potential for meaningful use in teaching and for realistic attainment by students. They were used meaningfully in programs of maternal and newborn health nursing at the Yale University School of Nursing and at the College of Nursing, University of Florida. These objectives specify that the student must give evidence, under a variety of circumstances, of her ability to:

1. Make explicit her purpose in nursing and the beliefs that she thinks give it validity.
2. Make appropriate application, within the realities of the existing learning situation, of knowledges and skills gained through her study of nursing and related disciplines.
3. Adapt the prescription for the patient's medical regimen in accordance with scientific principles and sound nursing and medical practices.
4. Respond to the patient's behavior in accordance with her intent and her purpose in nursing.
5. Make appropriate use, in her care of patients, of such resources as evaluation, comfort, support and therapeutic measures, as well as the facilities of the hospital, health agency, family and/or community.
6. Specify the reasons upon which her decision to take nursing action is based and justify it in light of her purpose in nursing and in accordance with scientific principles and sound nursing and medical practices.
7. Work with patients and their families and with other health workers in accordance with her purpose in nursing.
8. Fulfill her commitments within the realities in the existing situation and accept responsibility for her recommendations and her actions, and the outcomes of each and/or both.
9. Delegate aspects of nursing care to others on the nursing team (or health team) with respect for the patient's welfare and in accordance with the agency's policies.
10. Record and/or report adequately, appropriately and economically, information about the patient's state, progress and care.
11. Seek help when the need for help is experienced.

12. Challenge, with respect for the one whom she may be challenging, policies or practices related to care of patients (or to her learning) which seem to her to defeat her purpose in nursing (or in learning).
13. Identify and describe the specific factors that promoted, supported or impeded achievement of the results that she desired to obtain through her action in nursing or in learning.

Commitment No. 3.
Formulation of plans for student learning

Planning takes time, thought, energy, imagination and determination. It is an important aspect of clinical teaching, for the greater the care with which plans for student learning are made, the more meaningful will the student's learning experience be. The value of careful planning is also reflected in the attitudes of the staff in the clinical area. Generally, the more the staff has contributed to the plans for the students' clinical experiences, the smoother will be the implementation of the plans and the warmer the staff's response to students and instructor when they reach the clinical area.

The process of planning for student learning involves finding answers to three distinct questions:

1. What needs to be planned?
2. What specific plans need to be made?
3. How can the plans best be implemented?

- **What needs to be planned?**

    1. The course of study essential for preparation for nursing in the particular clinical specialty.
    2. The volume and variety of clinical experience desired for students.
    3. The instructor's own preparation for directing her students' clinical experiences.
    4. The background preparation students will need for their learning experiences in the clinical area.

5. The students' time schedule with respect to their learning experiences in the clinical area.
6. The system for evaluating students' progress in the particular course of study.
7. The nursing staff's participation in the clinical teaching program.
8. The teaching staff's responsibilities, distribution and time schedules, with respect to the students' learning experiences.

- What specific plans need to be made?

- - Course of study

To learn to function with security and competence in the clinical area, the student needs to assimilate, concurrently with her clinical experience, a body of theoretic, substantive and practical knowledge. Although its assimilation is enhanced by experience, the student may feel less at a loss when starting out in the clinical area if she has opportunity to gain at least some of this knowledge before she actually begins her clinical practice.

The instructor usually has the responsibility for making the plans for the course. Before she can do so meaningfully, however, she needs to know what courses and experience the students have already had. She also needs to know what resources in the community, the hospital, the school of nursing, and the educational institution with which the school is associated she can draw on to augment her students' classroom and clinical experiences.

In setting up a course of study, it is essential to plan for:

1. The scope of the course.
   Will it cover mostly normal processes, abnormal processes or both?
   Will it emphasize medical aspects of the clinical specialty, nursing aspects or both?
   Will it include theory and concepts relevant to the clinical specialty?

Will it include portions of such other disciplines as philosophy, the behavioral or social sciences?
2. The length of the course.
How many weeks will it run?
How many sessions will be held?
How long will each session be?
3. The content of the course.
What subject matter will be covered?
What will be the subject of each session?
What textbooks will be used?
What collateral reading will be suggested?
Will periodic, midterm and/or final examinations be given?
What assignments will be given?
Will students be expected to develop some sort of project?
4. The teaching participants.
Will teaching be carried out by one or more clinical instructors having the same clinical specialty, or by a team?
What sessions will each participating instructor teach?
Will students have opportunity to lead some sessions? If so, which ones?
Will any sessions be conducted by other clinical nursing specialists and by members of other disciplines such as anatomist, physician, pathologist, geneticist, social worker, nutritionist, psychologist or philosopher? If so, how many? By whom? When?
5. The format of the sessions.
Will they be conducted in the form of lectures, seminars, discussions or other?
Will visual aids be used? If so, what ones? When? How?
6. The time schedule.
When, in relation to onset of the clinical experience, should classes be started?
When can classes be held with respect to such considerations as available classrooms? other school commitments of students? clinical experience schedule? availability of others, who have agreed to participate in the teaching program?

Answers to such questions can guide the instructor in formulating her course of study. The best laid plans, though, "gang aft a-gley," and so may those for a course of study. A certain instructor may not be available on a particular day as planned, or some unforeseen happening in the clinical area may necessitate discussion in class of a subject not planned for. Such contingencies may occur at any time, and the instructor needs to recognize that changes in course plans will often have to be made. The plan should be regarded as a *guide*, not as an immutable set of directions.

• • **Student experience**

The volume and variety of clinical experience that can be arranged for students depends on the instructor's objectives for student learning and on the realities in the clinical situation. She has a wide choice, as a rule, for patients are apt to have emotional and social needs in addition to their physical, medical and nursing needs. The instructor who is clear about the kind of experiences she desires her students to have is usually able to find ways of providing them. This, however, calls for resourcefulness, adaptability and ingenuity in planning.

The type of clinical area or health service selected for student learning—medical, surgical, pediatric, obstetric or psychiatric—depends on the level of clinical study in which the student is currently engaged. If she is a beginning student, her first clinical experience may be on a medical unit, in a well-baby clinic or on a postpartum unit in the obstetric department. If she is a senior, she may be assigned to an intensive care unit or the operating room. The complexity of treatments and procedures with which she will be involved and the responsibilities she is expected to assume generally increase as she progresses in the school or in a particular clinical course. They vary, too, from unit to unit, but so far as actual nursing is concerned, the same responsibilities obtain in all clinical areas: 1) to identify the patient's need for help; 2) to minister the help needed; and 3) to validate that the patient's experienced need for help was met.

For the student to develop proficiency in carrying out these responsibilities, she must have, first and foremost, the chance to *care for patients*. Every patient, regardless of the illness that besets him, is unique. His problems, be they physical, physiological, mental, emotional or spiritual, are peculiar to him, and he has his own way of manifesting and experiencing them. Not only do the responses of each patient differ from those of every other patient, but they differ in themselves according to time and circumstances. Therefore, by insuring that the student will care for patients, the instructor will provide her with opportunities to become introduced to the manifestations of a variety of diseases, disorders and conditions, and to develop the three most basic of nursing skills: meaningful approaches, purposeful responses and resourceful action. Implicit in these basic skills are competencies in observation and communication, and in the implementation of various appropriate procedures.

Observation is an innate power that may be described as the energized ability to use one's own sensory organs; in other words, the ability to see, hear, feel, smell and taste. As a skill, however, it has a broader meaning, for, in this context, it includes the ability to make discriminating distinctions of what is sensed, to compare what is distinguished with one's concept of what is normal and expected, and to make plausible assumptions about the significance of the result of the comparison. For example, a nurse uses her power of observation when she notices that a patient winces when he uses his left arm. Her concept of normal arm use is movement unaccompanied by a wincing gesture. She may assume, therefore, that his left arm hurts when he moves it, and that there is something wrong with it. Thus, in the context of a skill, observation constitutes a constellation of mental exercises that may lead to awareness of inconsistencies in the immediate environment. Such a skill is important to nursing because the existence of inconsistencies may be suggestive of a problem that gives rise to a patients' need for help. Unlike the *power* of observation, however, the *skill* of observation is not an innate quality. It must be learned and developed—a fact that the instructor will need to consider when planning her students' experiences in the clinical area.

Communication may be verbal or nonverbal and may be carried out by word, look or manner. It is an art all of itself, one to which consideration undoubtedly was given in several of the student's earlier courses in the school. Ability to communicate meaningfully within the realities of a particular clinical area, however, adds a practical dimension to the student's learning of the art. It entails eliciting and giving meaningful responses during the student's involvement with patients. This may be direct involvement with the patients themselves; or it may be indirect involvement, on behalf of patients, with such others as members of patients' families, visitors, fellow students, members of the nursing heirarchy, doctors, other hospital personnel, community health and welfare workers or the instructor. To communicate purposefully, appropriately, adequately and economically with any one of these, represents a learning achievement vital to effective nursing. Consequently, in planning a student's experience, the instructor may want to give thought to situations that will afford the student opportunity to develop her ability to communicate meaningfully not only with the patient but with other individuals as well.

In addition to skills in observation and communication, effective nursing entails deft and timely application of measures that are inherent in the appropriate procedures. Dexterity is important in such application and can, of course, be acquired through repetitive practice in a non-clinical situation. Within the realities of a clinical area, however, implementation of procedures also requires the nurse to exercise judgment with respect to timeliness, appropriateness, adequacy and economy. Such judgment can best be developed in reality situations where demands are many and the need to make astute decisions exists. The realities differ in the various clinical areas. They differ also from minute to minute in any one clinical area. It is they that impose the need for the exercise of judgment in the execution of procedures. Thus, in planning students' experience, the instructor will need to consider not only the procedural needs of the patients and the competency needs of the individual student, but also the realities in the situation that may necessitate the exercise of judgment by the student.

Although it often is said that "experience is the best teacher," it may be more accurate to say that "thinking about one's experience is the best teacher." Learning is a post-experience phenomenon, but only if the student thinks about the experience, tries to reconstruct its salient features, evaluates the outcome and then attempts to identify the factors that brought about the results that she obtained from what she did. Thus, plans for student learning in clinical courses can be considered complete only if, along with everything else, they insure that each student will have opportunity to think about her experience analytically and to discuss it objectively and constructively with the instructor or her surrogate.

• • Preparation of the instructor for her students' clinical experience

Although the instructor may be a highly competent practitioner of nursing, when she is new to a clinical area she is apt to have misgivings about her ability to be as helpful to her students as she would like to be. To be sure, her orientation to her responsibilities undoubtedly included an introduction to the clinical supervisor and a meaningful conference with her, introductions to other unit personnel, a tour of the unit, and an explanation of a written statement of policies and routine procedures relating to practices on the unit. Although such orientation is helpful, it usually is not sufficient to give the instructor confidence in her ability to fulfill her responsibilities to her students when they are in the area. To develop such a sense of security before her students' arrival, she may decide to spend some time in the area as a staff nurse.

To arrange for such experience, the instructor will need to consider when she can best fit it into her schedule and when the head nurse can best tolerate having her, as a staff nurse, in the area. This last is particularly important because the instructor not only will need to be oriented to details of the service, but she can also anticipate making many requests for information about such things as where supplies are located, how to carry out special procedures, which doctor to call when a patient may be in distress, how to find information on the charts or even how to decipher some of the hieroglyphics and abbreviations she may find on the charts.

In addition, the instructor will also need to consider how much time she may require for this experience and what time of day would be best for her to be in the clinical area. So much usually goes on in the area, and so much about it may be different from what the instructor has been accustomed to, that she may need several exposures before she can find her way around the area readily and become familiar with patients, practices and personnel. Regarding the time of day, the instructor will find it helpful to begin at the beginning—when the night nurse gives the morning report to the day staff. Attendance at morning report will not only give her opportunity to learn of patients' problems and of occurrences in the area during the night, but also to gain impressions of attitudes and concerns about patients and reponsibilities individual nurses may display, of the volume of work to be done, of the method by which assignments are made, and of the status of intra-staff relationships. Attendance at morning report alerts the nursing staff to the fact of the instructor's presence and gives her a chance to tell them why she is there and to enlist their interest not only in responding to her needs for help, but also to those of her students when they arrive in the area.

• • **The students' preparation for clinical experience**

Whether she is a basic undergraduate student or a graduate student who has not practiced in the clinical setting for several years, the student approaching her first exposure to nursing in a certain clinical area may envision herself assuming responsibilities that are awesome and frightening. In a sense, she is justified in being apprehensive, for she will be caring for sick people who are in the hospital to get well and who expect a nurse to be understanding, knowledgeable, helpful and skillful. The student may worry about how to approach a patient, how to carry out some painful or embarrassing procedure or how to be helpful. She may also feel anxious about how the staff will respond to her and how she can come up to their expectations as well as to her own and those of her instructor. When such anxieties are present, they can seriously interfere with the student's ability to learn and to function competently in the clinical area. They need to be dispelled and, to a large degree they can be, if plans for the student's preparation for the clinical experience are made and carried out in advance. Preparation for her clinical experience may be obtained through demonstrations, individual or group conferences, rehearsals for practice within the realities, tours of the clinical area and informative written material. Some of these means may be more appropriate than others, but all have potential value; the instructor will want to give thought to what each may contribute as well as entail, and how she might make it of greatest use to the student.

• • • **Individual conferences**

These can provide opportunity for students to reduce their apprehensions, to gain encouragement and possibly suggestions, and to discuss pertinent questions raised by either the student or the instructor. Planning for them involves thought about their content, selection of a place in which to hold them, and setting a mutually satisfactory time.

• • • **Group conferences**

These may be utilized to save time in giving two or more students specific information about the clinical area, its staff and patients, and about the conduct expected of students with respect to staff members, instructor and patients; for demonstrating special procedures or devices in common use in the area; and for discussing questions of general interest.

• • • **Rehearsal for practice within the realities**

This is an excellent medium through which a student may be helped to alleviate any anxiety she may have about her ability to communicate meaningfully with patients and others in the clinical area. It provides, in a simulated clinical setting, opportunity for her: 1) to approach a "patient" or a "member of the staff" and to respond, without fear that she might commit a damaging or irreversible blunder with a real patient or staff member; 2) to gain an idea of the feelings a patient may have when he is approached or responded to by the nurse; 3) to express her own reactions to her way of functioning and make suggestions about what she might, perhaps, have said or done to obtain better results; and 4) to hear peers' as well as her instructor's comments and suggestions regarding what she said or did and what she might have said or done. In planning for rehearsals, the instructor needs to think about how to get students to want to participate in them, when to hold them and how to conduct them.

• • • A tour

A tour through the clinical area where the student will be may enable her to enter her experience with a degree of confidence that comes from familiarity with one's surroundings. This confidence will be further enhanced if she meets members of the nursing staff, especially the head nurse and/or team leader, and is introduced to members of the medical staff and such other personnel as the ward secretary, the aides and the kitchen maid. Planning for a tour will involve scheduling the time, deciding upon its scope, and notifying members of the nursing and medical staffs and other personnel that the tour will be held and that they may be asked to take part in it.

• • • Informative written material

This helps to reinforce the spoken word. It may also serve as a reminder to the student of what she is expected to do and to know. It often gives a student a sense of security, too, for she may be all too aware that she did not hear all of the information that was given orally at the time of the initial group conference. Included on an information sheet might be such items as:

1. Names of the members of the nursing, medical, secretarial and administrative staffs in the clinical area and the positions held by each.

2. Name of the instructor (s) in the area, her (their) role (s) and her (their) availability.
3. Name of the person to whom the student will report "on duty" and "off duty," when/if ill or in an emergency.
4. What is expected of students with respect to promptness, dress and grooming.
5. Written assignments to be fulfilled.
6. Time and place of conferences.
7. Suggested reading lists.
8. Courtesies and responsibilities to observe when visiting a patient at other than clinical experience time.
9. Measures the instructor will use to assess students' progress.

All such preparatory plans for students' clinical experience involve not just the instructor and students but also the clinical nursing staff. Place and time are especially important considerations, since some clinical units are busier than others and their involvements vary according to the day and the time of day. When and where conferences are to be held and who on the staff might participate in them are of real concern to the head nurse. When tours are to be conducted, how extensive they are to be, and who on the staff might be asked to take part in them are of concern to her, too. Rehearsals for practice will be meaningful only if rules for carrying them out are carefully established. The content of the information sheet will be of greater value if it includes suggestions from the clinical nursing staff. The instructor who respects the responsibilities carried by the nursing staff in the clinical area and also the contribution that members of the nursing staff can make to her teaching program, will consult with the head nurse and others on the staff without fail. This will not only help to engender a cooperative relationship between instructor and clinical nursing staff, but it also does much to enhance the quality of the students' experience in the clinical area.

• • Students' time schedule

Although the length of time that the students will be in any one clinical department is usually determined by the school's curriculum committee, the distribution of the students within the department and of their time in each of its areas is the responsibility of the clinical instructor. If, for example, the curriculum committee specifies that students should spend eight weeks in the department of obstetrics (40 days, actually), the instructor's distribution of students and their time might be: three days for orientation of all students; ten days for X number of students in the antepartum and postpartum clinics; ten days for X number in the labor and delivery rooms; ten days for X number in the rooming-in area; five days for X number in the conventional postpartum area; and two days for X number in the central nursery.

Providing for each student's rotation through all areas of a unit may present a planning problem since the number of students needing a particular experience at a particular time may exceed the number of patients in that special setting. In such an instance, the instructor may be able to make use of other facilities. For example, she may substitute experience in a physician's office for that in the clinics. Making such a change, however, may raise other planning problems such as how to accommodate the time of a few students, as well as that of the instructor, to the physician's office hours.

The instructor must also carefully plan which hours of the day the students will be in the clinical area. Factors she needs to consider in this connection are:

1. The kind of experience desired for the students. If, for example, a student needs experience in identifying and meeting patients' needs for help, morning or evening hours may be the best time for her to be on the service; while if, for some reason, she needs experience in meeting members of patients' families, it may be best for her to be on the unit during visiting hours.

2. The availability of instructional help. From a learning standpoint, clinical experience will be of greatest benefit to the student when she has ready access to an instructor for help when she needs it. Therefore, the times when an instructor can be in the clinical area is an important consideration in planning the students' hour schedules. Because of other than teaching commitments, the instructor is usually more able to fit herself into a daytime schedule than into an evening or night-time one. If, for some reason, she cannot be in the clinical area when her students are assigned to be there, she may be able to enlist the head nurse's aid in providing essential instruction and help. This usually presents no problem if the instructor has previously given the head nurse a list of the students' names along with a statement about what educational experiences they have already had, has kept her informed and has consulted with her about teaching plans, and has obtained her consent to give a helping hand should it be needed.
3. The need for continuity of service to patients. Although many times patients respond immediately to a nurse's ministrations, they frequently have more serious needs that are not so easily met. A little boy, for instance, may dread the operation scheduled for the next morning and wish that his nurse could go with him to the operating room, or at least see him off. Another patient may be acutely ill and withdrawn, and respond only minimally to the nurse as she gives him morning care. A newly delivered mother may recall the breast discomfort she experienced after her first child was born and dread the onset of lactation two or three days hence. Existing problems, such as those suggested by the behavior of any of these patients, can usually be resolved only over a period of time, often only at specific times. Generally, the nurse who has established a relationship with the patient is the one most likely to uncover the patient's need for help, and the one most desired by the patient to meet it.

Continuity of service by a particular nurse is important to many patients. It is also of special importance to the nurse, be she a student or a graduate. The enduring satisfactions in nursing come, to a large degree, from opportunities the nurse has to meet the challenge of a particular patient's problem and to give that patient meaningful service. For this reason, and because many times the nurse must have contact with a patient over a period of several days in order to help him resolve his problem, the instructor may need to consider—when planning her students' time in the clinical setting—ways of insuring opportunity for the student to care for a patient on several, preferably consecutive, days. In some instances, too, it is important to make provision for a student to visit, at home, a patient for whom she had cared while he was in the hospital.

4. The clinical area's involvements. Although the degree of activity obtaining on a service unit at any period of the day cannot be precisely foretold, it may be known to be greater on some days than others and, in some areas, considerable differences in involvement are known to exist between days, evenings and nights. On a Monday morning, for example, the medical unit of almost any hospital is apt to be a bustling place. Nurses are caring for patients, head nurses are familiarizing themselves with new developments relating to patients' needs, staffing and directives; technicians are getting specimens of one kind or another; doctors are making rounds; laundrymen are delivering linen; orderlies are moving beds or mopping floors. At night, however, relative quiet may prevail on a medical unit. On the other hand, nights may be the hectic times in the emergency room of the ambulatory service, while days, though busy, may progress at a steadier pace.

A student usually learns best when she can concentrate on what she is doing, but concentration can be difficult in an atmosphere of hustle, bustle, seeming confusion and, possibly, short-temperedness. Nevertheless, she will sometimes be caught up in such situations. They are part of the realities in nursing and, although they can be traumatic if experienced by a student before she is ready to cope with them, they also have valuable learning potential that the instructor often wants to exploit. In planning the schedule of hours when students will be in a particular clinical area, therefore, the instructor may want to consider not only its times of greatest pressure but also her objectives for her students' learning, the stage of the students' development in nursing, and her own availability to the students.

5. The number of staff nurses and other students in the area. The size of the nursing staff in a clinical area is apt to be greater some days than others—on week days, for example, as opposed to weekends and holidays. It may also vary according to day, evening or night. Consequently, staffing is a factor for the instructor to consider when planning her students' time schedules. Of course, it is important for students to be willing and ready to "pitch in and help out" occasionally when circumstances on the unit warrant it. But should the area be seriously understaffed continuously, repeated service demands could cause students undue stress, jeopardize their learning, and thwart the instructor in the attainment of her objectives.

Another factor for the instructor to take into account is the time when other students may be in the area. Some clinical settings provide experience for graduate students, basic nursing students, affiliating nursing students, and students in practical nursing programs. Should all or several of these different groups be in the clinical area at the same time, competition for experiences could be keen; students' learning might be impaired by their instructors' conflicts of interests; patients' goals could be defeated by the various students' learning needs; and the nursing staff's plans for patient care could be completely wrecked. Such a situation can be obviated if the instructor arranges with the head nurse for her students to

have experience in the area at times when only a few of the other students—or none of them—are there.
6. Students' need to attend classes. Classes which students are expected to attend are usually scheduled during daytime hours. Problems arise, however, when classes are held on days that the students are in the clinical area and they must leave unfinished what they may be doing with or for a patient in order not to be late or to miss a class. By implication, such interruption of a student's patient care activity may place higher value on her class attendance than on the completion of her clinical nursing assignment; and this, understandably, not only can be disconcerting to student, nursing staff and patient, but it is apt to defeat, irreversibly, the instructor's objective for student learning. Such a predicament may be avoided if the instructor plans the time when her students are to be in the clinical area *in relation to* their class schedule, not *around* it.
7. Inclusion of pre- and post-experience conferences. Some instructors recognize pre- and post-experience conferences as important parts of students' clinical experience and include time for them in their clinical time schedules. The pre-experience conference, for which as much as a half-hour may be allowed, is generally used to discuss and make plans for the students' ensuing activities. The post-experience conference needs to be longer. Students should have sufficient time to reconstruct the clinical experiences they have just had, to examine together, objectively and analytically, what they did and, hopefully, to envision with perspective the strengths and weaknesses in their nursing practice. Such conferences add an important learning dimension to the students' clinical experiences, but unless provision is made for them on the students' time schedules, they can easily be overlooked.

All these factors suggest that the students' time schedule represents a powerful instrument for promoting student education and for cementing faculty-nursing staff relationships. It influences attitudes, morale and learning and, consequently, it needs to be seriously and thoughtfully planned.

• • **Evaluation of student participation in a program of clinical nursing education**

Evaluation of a student's participation in a program of clinical nursing education is one of the most difficult—and possibly the most resisted—of the responsibilities the clinical instructor faces. The educational institution, be it school, college or university, may specify a scoring (grading) system that the instructor is to use; for example, Honors, High Pass, Pass and Fail, or the symbols A, B, C, D and E, or even the familiar numerical grading scale that runs from 100 down to 0. Such specification, however, is seldom accompanied by an interpretation of the symbols as indicators of levels of quality of the student's learning. Consequently, the instructor is expected to convert the student's functioning, in relation to the various learning opportunities that are provided for her, into a quantitative measure indicative of the student's progress toward attainment of proficiency in her course of study. This responsibility vests considerable power in the instructor. At the same time, any strain that may exist in the instructor-student relationship may be heightened by the fact that grades given by the instructor are usually accepted by the school administrators without serious question, and that they are used not only as qualitative measures of what the student has learned, but also as bases for the student's eligibility to be promoted within the school or graduated from it.

One may reasonably assume that the clinical instructor's desire is to discharge her grade-giving responsibility with objectivity, reliability and validity. She recognizes that the grades she gives may exert a strong influence both on the student's progression through the school and on her acceptability as a candidate either for continued education or for employment of a kind the student might wish. The problem, however, is how to insure a high degree of fairness in giving them. An answer may be found in careful planning that includes:

• • • **The provision of numerous and varied opportunities for the student to disclose her thinking and her competence in dealing with the realities in her learning situation**

The instructor needs tangible evidence of a student's progressive ability to grasp concepts and to apply them meaningfully within the realities of the clinical situation. Her concern is the thinking process that underlies the student's judgment as well as the skill that the student displays in the actions she takes. Thus, self-disclosure devices that she may set up for her students might include recitations and classroom presentations, involvement in care of patients, written reconstructions of selected nursing experiences, individual conferences, group conferences or classes, weekly written summaries of the students' thinking about their learning experiences, term papers, progress tests and examinations.

• • • **The provision of opportunities to gain first-hand knowledge of how the student thinks and functions**

For the instructor to find out how the student thinks and functions, she will have to maintain close contact with her and make her own assessment of the student's responses to whatever self-disclosure devices have been set up. This does not rule out the possibility that other members of the faculty may also make assessments of the student's responses. Indeed, the possibility of bias may be reduced when more than one instructor makes such assessments, and the results are compared and possibly even reconciled.

• • • **The specification of desirable student attributes and their behavioral manifestations**

Desirable student attributes epitomize the characteristics that the instructor believes are the hallmarks of a qualified practitioner of nursing. They derive from her system of professional values and are reflected in the objectives that she has set up for the course she is teaching. In specifying them, she enunciates a set of qualities that she expects the student to display

Sample Set of Desirable Student Attributes and Their Behavioral Manifestations

Attribute	Behavioral Manifestations
Constancy in purpose:	Keeps to point and holds direction. Acts in accordance with intent. Seeks clarification of evident discrepancies.
Understanding:	Acts with apparent awareness of actual or potential implications, effects or results of her actions. Responds supportively to others' needs, feelings or situations. Evidences grasp of facts and/or knowledge, and/or concepts.
Competence:	Applies concepts pertinently in practice. Observes details; acts with accuracy. Seeks help in context of existing realities.
Deliberateness:	Validates assumptions before acting. Particularizes individuals and situations. Gives valid reasons for affirmations and/or actions.
Responsibleness:	Fulfills commitments with consideration for all others. Economizes in use of own and/or others' time and property. Tempers praise or criticism with constructive comments or suggestions.
Resourcefulness:	Improvises safely and with imagination. Varies approach to people and problems in context of existing realities. Makes judicious use of existing means and facilities.

in ever increasing degree as she progresses through the course, and she lets others—including the student—know what she values in a professional practitioner. Since behavioral manifestations are observable and thus measurable, such a set of qualities can be converted into a tool for evaluating the student's performance and progress.

The sample set (see page 46) of desirable student attributes and their behavioral manifestations is a simplified version of one that has been used in evaluating students' participation in a program of clinical nursing education. It may have meaning for other instructors if they can fashion it into a tool for their own use by examining it, refining it, trying it out, and then improving on it on the basis of their experience with it.

• • • **The construction of a system of symbols for use as qualitative measures of the attributes**

Symbols used to designate the degree to which a student has manifested the desirable attributes in her participation in course or in a school's educational program may be words, letters or numbers. Words sometimes used are Excellent, Very Good, Good, Fair, Fail; Honors, High Pass, Pass, Fail; or even just Pass, Fail. Letters may be A,B,C,D,E, with A being comparable to Excellent or Honors, and E comparable to Fail. Numbers may range anywhere from 100 down to 0, with 100 signifying Excellent and lower numbers scaling downward to and below Fail.

The number of symbols used varies according to school policies which may also dictate the quantitative value to be attached to each word or letter symbol. Thus, Excellent may symbolize a value anywhere from 95 to 100 on a 0-100 scale, and Fail may indicate any grade below 60. The point of demarcation between Pass and Fail is generally an arbitrary one. Some schools use 60 as the turning point, some 65, and some 70. In addition, school policy may specify the number of C or D grades that a student may be allowed to have in combination with a designated number of A's or B's on her final report without jeopardizing her eligibility for promotion or graduation.

In specifying the symbols to use, along with their values in terms of Pass or Fail, a school provides the clinical instructor with a grade system that it apparently considers functional. The instructor, however, needs to give it meaning in terms of her students' learning. This means that she needs to develop her own evaluative tool for measuring the quality of her students' behavioral manifestations of how they think and function as a result of their clinical instruction and, after applying it to her students' learning, translate the resultant scores into the school's grade system. If the instructor has given consideration in her planning to such steps as those that are suggested on page 45, she may be able to make such translation with a high degree of consistency and a reasonable degree of objectivity.

• • • **The assignment of a numerical value—absolute and range—as a basis for computing the composite value of the quality of a student's desirable attributes as manifested in a particular learning situation**

A learning situation constitutes a student's experience in a class, conference or clinical area, her execution of a written assignment or reconstruction of a nursing incident, or her performance in an examination. In the course of any of these activities, she has opportunity to manifest various aspects of desirable attributes that she may possess. For example, she may be meticulous in carrying out the details of a nursing care assignment but be grudging in her response to co-workers' needs, hence a high value symbol would be accorded her for Competence, and a relatively low one for Understanding. It is the composite of such assigned values that suggests the quality of her total participation in that particular learning situation. The numerical equivalents of letter or word symbols used to denote degree of quality must be specified so that they may be totalled and an average established. Numbers lend themselves to averaging; letters or words do not. What numerical equivalent—absolute and range—an instructor may wish to assign to a letter or word symbol, is usually an arbitrary decision. In general, she may find it easier to work with small whole numbers than with large or fractional ones; and she may want to take into consideration

REALITIES

the number of symbols used, the number of attributes to be measured and the range of the fail area.

To illustrate:

If the five letter symbols A, B, C, D and E are used in evaluating the six suggested attributes, the numerical equivalents might be:

  A = 10 Range: 9+ through 10
  B = 7   " 6+ " 9
  C = 5   " 4+ " 6
  D = 3   " 3   " 4
  E = 1   " 1 up to 3

In this system, the point of demarcation between Pass and Fail is just below 3; and the range of the Fail area is from 1 to 3.

On the other hand, should only four letter symbols be used in evaluating the student's manifestation of the six attributes, the numerical equivalents might be:

  A = 4 Range: $3\frac{1}{2}$ through 4
  B = 2   "   2 up to $3\frac{1}{2}$
  C = 1   "   1 up to 2
  D = −1 "   −1 up to 1

In this system, the point of demarcation between Pass and Fail is just below 1 and the range of the Fail area is from −1 up to 1.

• • • **Construction of a form on which to score, for every learning situation, a symbol signifying the degree to which the student manifested, in relation to it, the designated desirable attributes**

In order to keep track of her estimate of the quality of a student's participation in any one learning situation, the instructor needs a score sheet on which to record her impression of the degree to which the student manifested, in what she did, the various desirable attributes. Such a score sheet should be simple in format, easy to use and adequately spacious. An explanation of how to use the form could be added as a footnote.

Course: _____ Student: _____
Semester: _____ Year: _____
(Title of university or school of nursing)
Score sheet for Evaluating Student Participation in Learning Situations

ATTRIBUTE	SCORE	Ed. Activity: _____ Date: _____
Constancy in Purpose		Substantiating facts:
Understanding		
Competence		
Deliberateness		
Responsibleness		
Resourcefulness		
Score, total av.		Instructor:

ATTRIBUTE	SCORE	Ed. Activity: _____ Date: _____
Constancy in Purpose		Substantiating facts:
Understanding		
Competence		
Deliberateness		
Responsibleness		
Resourcefulness		
Score, total av.		Instructor:

ATTRIBUTE	SCORE	Ed. Activity: _____ Date: _____
Constancy in Purpose		Substantiating facts:
Understanding		
Competence		
Deliberateness		
Responsibleness		
Resourcefulness		
Score, total av.		Instructor:

Directions for scoring:

Score Symbols:

The instructor may need to experiment with a variety of formats before she is able to decide which is the most useful for her. One that was found workable when used to evaluate students' participation in a course in maternity nursing is presented here as a sample.

• • • **Summarization of students' scores at specified intervals**

A clinical nursing course comprises a number of different learning situations that the student may experience over a specified number of days, weeks or even months. Hopefully, the quality of her participation, as reflected by the way she manifests designated desirable attributes in what she does, will improve steadily as she progresses in the course. The instructor needs to know, at all times, how the student is progressing and what

Graphic Record of Composite Scores

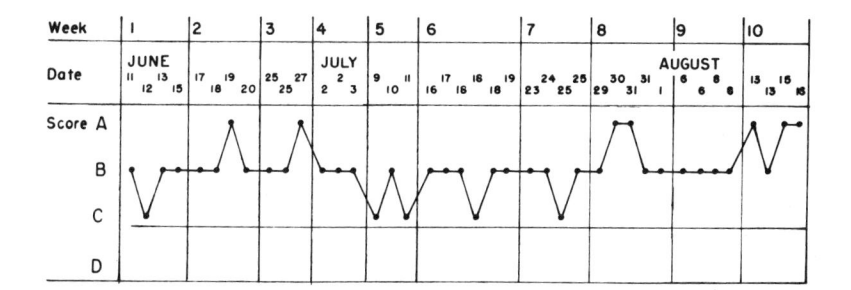

Week	1	2	3	4	5	6	7	8	9	10
Date	JUNE 11 13 12 15	17 19 18 20	25 27 25	JULY 2 3	9 11 10	17 16 19 16 18	24 25 23 25	30 31 29 31 1	AUGUST 6 8 6 8	13 15 13 15

Score A, B, C, D (graphic line plot)

Graphic record of composite scores indicating the quality of a graduate student's participation in learning activities during the first 10 weeks of a clinical nursing course. Activities scored were classes; individual conferences; clinical experience including tutorial practice; rehearsals for practice; reconstructions of nursing incidents; and summaries of thinking. Clinical experience was introduced during the fifth week and was continued through the eighth week.

progress she has made. She can achieve this awareness by summarizing the student's scores at regular intervals. Such summaries will also reveal the student's strengths or weaknesses with respect to desirable attributes that influence the quality of her work. The student's strengths, weaknesses and progress may be brought into still sharper focus by graphically charting the scores. The resultant chart (see sample) may then be used as a basis for discussing with the student the quality of her participation in the course.

• • • The provision for opportunity to discuss a student's scores with her at stated intervals, or on request, with willingness to revise them should the student present valid reasons for the instructor's doing so

By allowing the student to see and challenge the scores assigned to the quality of her participation in the various learning situations, the instructor shows that she recognizes the fact that the meaning to the student of the behavior evaluated may be different from its meaning to the instructor. Of necessity, the instructor assigns scores according to her assumptions based on her perceptions of the student's behavior in the context of the realities of which the instructor is aware. Thus, the scores are based on a unilateral decision and this militates against unbiased evaluations. When the student has a chance to present her reasons for having taken a certain action, the instructor's perception of the situation may be broadened and she may gain new insights that will justify her in revising or modifying the scores. The student's perception of the situation may also be broadened, and this may lead to clearer understanding and acceptance of the scores.

• • Participation of nursing staff in the clinical teaching program

The nursing staff can be a staunch ally of the instructor in her actual teaching. Their participation, whether incidental or formal, is essential, and deserves respect as well as recognition in the instructor's plans for student learning.

Incidental participation entails responses to students' on-the-spot questions and to their requests for information or for

REALITIES

some form of help. Formal participation refers to the special sessions that designated members of the clinical nursing staff may conduct or in which they may take part. Such sessions include orientation to the area, demonstrations of use of special equipment or of "set-ups" for such therapeutic measures as surgery, delivery or treatments, and conferences on special care of particular patients. In planning for the nursing staff's participation, the instructor may want to give the head nurse a list of the students' names and some background information about each of them. She may discuss with her how best to alert the nursing staff to the fact that the students are coming to the area so that they will be prepared for the numerous incidental demands the students will inevitably make of them. Together, they will need to make arrangements for the formal teaching sessions—when and where they will be held, how and by whom they will be conducted, what their content will be, and which members of the staff will attend them.

In addition to making all these plans, the instructor and the head nurse may talk about the staff's responsibility with respect to the students, both when the instructor is in the clinical area and when she is not. They may discuss, for instance, what a staff member might do, should she become aware of something a student may have omitted doing or of an error she committed; and whether a staff member may, without first consulting the instructor, change some phase of the student's assignment in order to let her take advantage of some special opportunity that arises unexpectedly and which she thinks would be of interest to the student. The head nurse may want to ask how often students are apt to be left on the unit without their instructor, what she may expect of them and what the instructor may expect of her. Such discussion can result in guidelines for cooperative working relationships between nursing staff and instructor and contribute meaningfully to the students' learning.

The instructor also may want to let the staff know that, at stated intervals, she would appreciate having their impressions of her students' capabilities in clinical practice. Their opinions, backed up by substantiating facts or experiences, can be valuable supplements to the instructor's impression of her students' progress.

• • The teaching staff's responsibilities and time schedule

Regardless of the size of the teaching staff for a particular clinical specialty, instructors' responsibilities are many and varied. Instructors occupy, in a sense, pivotal positions between the student and the clinical nursing staff; between the student and other clinical personnel (medical, attending and house staff, social workers, nutritionists, to name a few); between the student and administrative nursing staff; and between student and nursing school dean or director. What the student does in the clinical area has implications for each of these people and groups. Consequently, the instructor, who is held accountable not only for her students' clinical activities but also for their progress, must take into consideration when she plans her clinical teaching program:

The students. In addition to planning for them a course of study involving a program of learning (classes, clinical experience, conferences, time schedules, reading lists and informative material of various kinds), she must also plan for evaluation of their progress.

The clinical nursing staff. In addition to planning for their participation in the clinical teaching, she must also plan for keeping them informed about essential developments or changes in the students' program and, at its end, for expression in writing of her appreciation for their help.

The other clinical personnel. She may need to consider how to alert them to the fact that students are coming to the clinical area, how to inform them about pertinent aspects of the students' educational backgrounds and activities, and whether to enlist their participation in the clinical teaching program and how they might participate.

The administrative nursing staff (supervisor and director). She may need to consider how to gain their approval of her plans for her students' activities in a particular clinical area, and how to keep them informed about significant developments or changes in the program.

REALITIES

The school administrative staff. She may need to formulate and think through plans for meeting the definite demands that the school, through its administrative staff, imposes on its instructors. These demands may include preparation of course outlines, schedules and reports, and sending copies of them to the school office at specified times; attendance at meetings of many kinds; and active membership in various school committees and those of local, state and national nursing and related organizations.

Developing a clinical teaching program is a multi-faceted undertaking. The instructor who is responsible for this task must not only think through all that is entailed in planning learning experiences for students, but she must also decide how the many functions of the program can be appropriately distributed among the teaching staff, how much time to allow for each activity, what days and hours of the day the various activities can best be carried out, and how she can appropriately thank the nursing staff and others who may collaborate in implementing the program.

- **How can implementation of the plans be assured?**

This is a question that the instructor would do well to explore in advance, since the fact of making plans does not insure that they will be carried out as intended. For example, the instructor may have planned with the head nurse for the students' orientation to the clinical unit at 10 A.M. on a designated Tuesday morning. When she and the students arrive on the unit at the appointed time, however, she finds that the head nurse is ill and off duty, and that she had forgotten to notify the relief nurse of the orientation plans.

The realities that obtain in the situation when implementation of plans is to be effected, determine the possibility of actualization. Although the instructor may assume that the realities will be supportive, the chance always exists that they will not be. The adage "there is many a slip 'twixt the cup and the lip" holds true for the best laid teaching plans. To insure against nonsupport by the realities, and to safeguard the implementation of her plans, the instructor needs to take three positive steps:

1. Establish priorities.
2. Confirm plans in writing.
3. Reconfirm plans just prior to time of implementation.

Examination of plans that have been formulated and committed to paper will reveal numerous tasks that must be undertaken in order to effect implementation. They cannot all be executed at the same time. By particularizing them, however, and ordering them according to their importance and time sequence, they will constitute a priority list that can be useful in three ways:

1. It can be checked and so insure that all necessary tasks will be carried out according to schedule.
2. It can give substance to a request for help, should plans be broader in scope than the instructor can implement alone.
3. It can serve as a basis for making assignments when two or more instructors are responsible for execution of plans.

The instructor usually arranges for implementation of her plans, either in conference or by telephone, with whomever is involved in them. It is wise to follow up such discussion with a letter or memorandum (keeping a carbon copy for her file), confirming the decisions. Such confirmation may clarify some aspect of the plan which possibly had not been heard or fully understood, and may have use as a reminder of decisions made, when the time comes for implementation of the plans. In addition, it might serve as a source of information for those who are not involved in the plans in the beginning but may become so, as did the nurse who took over for the ill head nurse in the example cited earlier.

Not only is it well to confirm decisions in writing, but it is also sound practice to reconfirm them just prior to the time for their implementation. This may be done by a telephone call or by a quick visit to the area or the office of the one involved. By doing this, the instructor may gain reasonable assurance that the realities are still supportive for her plans. If they are, implementation may proceed. However, should unforeseen circumstances have altered the anticipated realities (illness of the head nurse, for example), the instructor may need to think through how she can change the plans and initiate the necessary adjustments.

Commitment No. 4.
Implementation of plans

A clinical instructor is assumed to be knowledgeable and competent. How knowledgeable and competent she is, however, is a matter of speculation on the part of her employer and can be ascertained only after the instructor has had opportunity to prove herself in the realities of the teaching situation. The instructor may expect—and may well ask—the employer to give her some idea of aspirations or plans that may have been made for development of the program. Then, by accepting appointment, the instructor commits herself to implement those plans through her teaching. To do this well, and in accordance with her central purpose in clinical teaching, she must have such special attributes as understanding, ability, motivation and energy. These four together constitute the dynamics that convert intent to implement plans into actual implementation.

Understanding signifies a mental grasp of subject matter in the context of its relevant relationships, involvements and implications and of the may subtleties at play within the realities of the existing situation. It derives from a broad spectrum of factual, speculative and practical knowledges that have been acquired through formal study, practice and associations, and have been tempered by meaningful experiences in life. It is not an innate quality, but almost every human being has the capacity to develop it to some degree. Understanding is an essential concomitant of clinical teaching. When the instructor possesses it to an appreciable degree, she is apt to have also developed the three companion qualities of wisdom, intelligence and sensitivity, all of which are indispensable to action needed to achieve desired results.

Ability is the faculty to function with competence in any particular situation. It is a confidence-producing quality, for it enables the one who has it to act with a high degree of sureness. It also fosters, in the recipient a willingness—even a sense of relief—to have what needs doing done by an able person. When the term is applied to a clinical instructor, the implication is that she is proficient in the practice of both teaching and nursing. It means, in other words, that she has developed and can apply the observational, procedural and communicative skills that are inherent in identifying needs-for-help, be they of student or of patient; in rendering help appropriately; and in validating that the help rendered was meaningful to student or patient and also consonant with her central purposes in clinical teaching and in nursing.

Motivation is a drive to act that lies dormant within each individual until aroused by an emotional, psychological or sensory response to some reality in a situation the individual has experienced, is experiencing or believes he may experience. Its roots lie within the individual's system of values and beliefs, and its strength is commensurate with his understanding of this system and the respect he accords it. Motivating factors or situations are legion. They may be straightforward and simple, or conflicting and complex as, for example, a smile, a threat, a word of praise, a cry of pain, a promise given or a feared event.

> An instructor tells herself at breakfast time, "I must call the head nurse first thing this morning, as I promised her I would, about the students' clinical experience in her area tomorrow." When she arrives at her office, she goes to the telephone and makes the call. In this instance, the instructor's recall of a promise given was the major motivating factor that sparked her energy and caused her to make the phone call. Such other factors as the imminence of the students' experience or the nature of plans she had made and her desire to have them work out well, undoubtedly added strength to the spark, but the dominant motive that caused

her to make the call "first thing this morning," was her promise to the head nurse. Suppose, on the other hand, that just as she arrived at her office, a secretary told her that an emergency faculty meeting had been called for 8:30 A.M. and that it was particularly important for her to attend it. This announcement startled her and raised the question in her mind, "What's up?" As other faculty members arrived, she speculated with them about the cause of the meeting. Minutes slipped by and soon 8:30 A.M. was at hand. Only then did she remember the telephone call she had promised to make, but that recollection was immediately overridden by the disquieting question, "Should I make it now?" If she did, she would be late to the meeting, and this could have unpleasant consequences; if she did not, she would be breaking her promise to the head nurse and this, too, could have unpleasant consequences.

Generally, the key to resolving such dilemmas lies within the instructor's value system. If, for example, the instructor in the situation described above believes that a promise imposes on her the obligation to keep it; if her philosophy incorporates the concept of "resoluteness to act dynamically in relation to her beliefs;" and if her central purpose in clinical teaching commits her to reconciling her assumptions about the realities with her purpose, then, in all probability, she will make the telephone call as promised, and risk the unpleasant consequences *she assumes* may result from her late arrival at faculty meeting. If, on the other hand, she is unable to bring her values clearly into focus, her motivation to make the phone call "now" may be submerged by the more impelling motive to arrive at the meeting on time.

Energy is the fuel which, when sparked by motivation, ignites the effort that must be exerted in order to get the job done. Some individuals are endowed with more of it than others, and some use it more liberally than others. Energy, coupled with motivation produces action and, when this coupling is done with understanding and ability, the action produced will result in implementation. However, like any fuel, energy needs to be used with judgment and care, for if applied too vigorously or in too great an amount, it can overwhelm or destroy; while if released too weakly or too tenuously, it can defeat by default.

The clinical instructor needs to be generously supplied with all four attributes. If she is weak in any one or all of them, she jeopardizes her entire program of clinical teaching. If she is strong in each, she has the potential for carrying out her plans with confidence, competence and enthusiasm.

Commitment No. 5.

Engagement in related activities that contribute to self-realization and to improvement of nursing practice

To maintain vitality in her teaching and to extend her usefulness beyond the educational community of which she is a part, the clinical instructor needs to complement her teaching with activities that are broadening, insight-producing and capable of contributing, directly or indirectly, to the improvement of her teaching and of nursing practice generally. Such activities include further study, purposeful clinical practice of nursing, nursing research and relevant writing for publication.

Before undertaking such complementary activities, however, the instructor needs to gain a degree of confidence in her own capability as a clinical teacher. It takes time to accumulate experience through which to develop and test her abilities sufficiently to give her that confidence. This is particularly true of the nurse who is new to the field of clinical teaching. As clinical instructor, she views the realities in changed perspective and is confronted by a new set of responsibilities. The patient becomes a subject for her *students'* care—not for care by her. Without taking over, she must facilitate the students' efforts to meet their patients' needs for help in accordance with their purposes in nursing. She also may need to plan the students' program of learning, arrange for implementation of the plans and participate in carrying them out. In addition, she has to learn her way about in the clinical area, the community, the school and university with their facilities and personnel. For the new instructor, an entire year may be needed in which to adjust to and become familiar with the many facets of her clinical teaching job, and a second year for her to become effective in it. When she has developed confidence in her ability and feels reasonably secure in her position of clinical instructor, then she may be ready to branch out and engage meaningfully in such related activities as further study, purposeful practice, nursing research and relevant writing for publication.

- **Further study**

The nurse instructor usually undertakes further study for one of three reasons: 1) to start work toward attainment of a higher degree; 2) to gain added knowledge; or 3) to exploit a special interest.

Often, part of the program leading to a higher degree, and sometimes all of it, may be undertaken on a fragmented basis, allowing the instructor to register for only one or two required or elective courses each term. Many universities, however, limit the number of years a student may take to complete the course work required for attainment of the degree. Consequently, once the instructor embarks on such part-time study, it is important for her to try to complete it as soon as possible. Her interest in doing so may be reinforced, too, by the importance that the academic world attaches to the degree. University schools of nursing, especially those offering graduate programs of study, usually require that nurses seeking appointment to their faculties have earned their Masters degrees, and eligibility for promotion, or sometimes even for continuation on the faculty beyond a specified time limit, may be dependent, in part, on the nurse-instructor's undertaking of doctoral study with serious intent to complete it. Thus, graduate study is of tangible economic value to the nurse-instructor. It is the intangibles that are gained in the process of earning the degree, however, that may contribute to the improvement of her teaching and through it, of nursing practice generally. Among these may be a broadening of academic, cultural and professional horizons; the realization of her own intellectual potential; formation of disciplined habits of inquiry and of study; deepened understanding of the complexities of life including the nature of man; and an enlarged capacity for meaningful service.

Each year, a growing number of universities and service agencies offer short-term courses in clinical or functional areas. These workshops, seminars or institutes, are open to qualified nurses who may or may not be clinical instructors. Many are held during the summer months. Titles of a few such courses that have been given include: Teaching in Medical-Surgical Nursing, (summer session); Science Principles Applied to Teaching and/or Clinical Nursing, (2-week workshop); Nursing Care of the Patient with Acute Myocardial Infarction, (2-week workshop); Curriculum, (4-day work conference); Family Mental Health, (4-week seminar); Nursing in Gerontology, (4-week seminar); Television and the Learning Process in Nursing, (3-day course). A number of these short courses are funded by grants from private foundations or public agencies for the express purpose of enabling those attending them to gain insights that will lead to enhancement of the quality of practice in clinical teaching or in nursing.

Clinical instructors also may have opportunity to enroll—not for credit but for interest, relaxation or enjoyment—in cultural courses offered by a university or by a school of arts and crafts. Such courses often are spiritually as well as intellectually satisfying and may influence the instructor's attitude in subtle but positive ways.

For many nurses, participation in programs of study of any kind is stimulating and enriching. It adds a new dimension to their thinking and at the same time provides them with resources that are permanently theirs and that they will draw upon, as time goes on, in countless, unexpected and unpredictable ways.

- **Purposeful practice of nursing**

Although the clinical instructor may spend much of her time in the clinical area, her focus, when there, is her students' functioning in the care of patients, not her own. However, in a world in which scientific and medical knowledge is rapidly expanding and the realities are constantly changing, the nurse's ways of functioning and responding must also change. Competencies developed in nursing experiences of yesterday may not be adequate in those of today, so that the clinical instructor who aims to keep her teaching meaningful and up-to-date may find it fruitful to periodically engage herself in some particular phase of clinical practice. She may be able to do this at specific periods of the day or week, or at a time of the school year when her teaching load is light. One instructor, for example, with little experience in caring for patients who are subjected to various kinds of monitors and other electronic devices, spent part of each weekend on the intensive care unit in order to learn about nursing procedures that involve the use of such devices. Another instructor, to deepen her understanding of maternity patients' hopes and fears and to increase her ability to meet the needs for help they may be experiencing, met once a week in conference with expectant mothers and made follow-up visits to each of them when they were hospitalized. Still another instructor, in order to develop understanding so that she could help her students resolve problems they were experiencing in a busy medical clinic, spent part of one semester as staff nurse in the clinic and gained valuable insights and ideas.

In addition to such specific reasons for undertaking nursing practice, the clinical instructor may involve herself in the care of patients for the pure pleasure of doing so, or for the lift to spirit and morale that a patient's appreciative responses can give. Whenever she does so, however, it is important that she make clear her intended change in function (from instructor to nurse) so that her associates on the nursing staff will understand why she is where she is and doing what she is doing, and will not only be accepting of her presence, but will give her essential support.

- **Nursing research**

Research is a form of inquiry that leads to new knowledge or, by testing presumed knowledge leads to its affirmation or negation. Research is not an end in itself. It functions as a developer or tester of theory that guides practice and which, when translated into practice, may improve it. Thus, research can indirectly contribute to the improvement of practice; and it will do so if the theory (concepts) it tests or develops has meaning for practice and is translated into it.

By virtue of her faculty position, the clinical instructor has a unique opportunity to do nursing research. She is free to come and go in the clinical area; she usually is privileged to spend as much time there as she desires; she need not become involved in service pressures and demands; and she may take time to observe and become aware of problems nurses seem to be experiencing in their care of patients. She can take time, too, to think about such problems, their manifestations, their possible causes, the common thread that may run through them and their apparent effects, to generalize them into a larger problem and then to conceptualize a way to resolve it. Such conceptualization constitutes the substance of theory which, when clearly articulated, may be subject for research.

The clinical instructor has a compelling reason to engage in research. As a nurse, her concern for patients' welfare may motivate her to try to solve problems experienced in nursing practice; but as a teacher of students of nursing, problem-solving that applies to the solution of a single problem only is not enough. She needs theories that will serve her students as guides to the kind of practice she deems good. Such theories are developed through practice and are tested and refined through research.

- **Relevant writing for publication**

Relevant writing for publication is a means by which ideas may be shared with a larger audience than is possible through face-to-face confrontations. Its great value, however, is that it may serve as a route to progress. Once articulated, written down and published, ideas, concepts and theories are given a degree of tangibility, and can be preserved as well as promulgated for purposes of reference, application, elaboration and development not only by contemporary readers but by future generations of readers as well.

The clinical instructor has a special stake in writing for publication. Her activities are designed to produce explicit results of a desired kind within the realities of existing and future situations. The very nature of her calling makes her sensitive to what is effective and what is ineffective in achieving desired results, and causes her to seek to develop better ways of attaining specific goals. Her ideas, concepts and ways of functioning may be accepted and applied by her students, and transmitted by them to others, but unless they have been preserved in published form, their identity may be altered in the process of transmission and become irretrievably lost. On the other hand, the publication of her ideas and concepts insures their preservation and inviolability. It also makes them available not only to her students, but also to her professional colleagues who may be seeking ways to improve their practice. By sharing her ideas in this tangible form, she enables them to help turn the wheels of progress. It is only when ideas can be examined that they can be apprehended; when they can be apprehended, they can be translated into practice; and when they are incorporated into practice, a better way of functioning may result.

• • • • • • • • • • • •

The Recipient: The Student*

The student is the recipient for whom a clinical teaching program is instituted. She may be presumed to have enrolled in such a program because she believes that it provides something she wants but does not have—specific knowledge, skills, abilities and understanding that will enable her to assume professional responsibilities in the future and to pursue a definite course of action acceptably, constructively and productively.

The road to learning, however, is often a rocky one—a fact that the student may not fully appreciate when she first embarks upon it. At the outset, after the excitement of convocation has subsided, she may find herself relegated to the position of "low man on the totem pole," one that may be hard to accept, especially if she had enjoyed prestige in school or college or had been engaged in responsible work of any kind. She may discover, too, as she progresses in the course, that she is expected to give full time to her studies and that she must drastically curtail the extra-school activities in which she has been —or would like to be—involved. She may also feel overwhelmed, on occasion, by class and clinical experiences and associated assignments that place heavy demands on her time and energy and which may be threatening to the image of herself that she may want to project. Although such experiences and assignments have been designed, as a rule, to stimulate her thinking and add depth to her understanding, they also have potential

---

* The feminine pronoun is used throughout this part of the book in the interest of simplicity. It does not imply lack of recognition that students may be either male or female.

for uncovering areas of uncertainty, ignorance and ineptitude that she might rather not recognize or have revealed. Then, as end of the academic year nears, the fear of not being able to complete requirements for either promotion or graduation may loom as a specter of increasing proportions. The anxieties attendant on any such circumstances have been known to seriously impair a student's ability to function adequately and to set up a vicious circle of discouragement and frustration.

Inherent in any educational program, thus, are tension-producing situations that the student may not have anticipated but with which she must learn to cope. This is particularly true of a program that is clinically oriented. In such a program, the student is expected not only to learn, but also to demonstrate, within the realities of life situations, that she has learned what she was expected to learn and can apply it meaningfully in giving nursing care to patients. Consequently, the instructor, in addition to providing opportunity for the student to develop resources of knowledge, insights and skills, may want to consider how to provide outlets through which the student may express her anxieties and channel them toward constructive resolution. One such outlet can be the weekly "summary of thinking" which students in some programs are asked to write. Frankness is encouraged. The students' identities are not revealed and the instructor responds to their comments in writing. In one such summary, a student commented on her effort to be "deliberate" in her nursing:

> So anxious was I, and am I, to be deliberate in my nursing—that is, to clarify and validate—that I would get upset with myself because I was not succeeding. Consequently, because of my rush and frustration, I blocked my own efforts. . . . After thinking about this, though, I believe if I just slow down, relax, use my head and quit pushing myself, that my understanding of how to be deliberate in my nursing may become much clearer.

Another student, describing insights she gained as a result of her frustration in the clinical area, wrote:

What frustrates me is my lack of continuity in using the process of nursing. I find myself assuming, making responses based on the assumptions, and ignoring my perceptions. I try to get the patient to do what I want her to do, which is not necessarily what is best for her, and I find myself rambling on in a conversation without any specific worthwhile purpose. Why? I think because I lack clarity in the purpose of nursing and skill in using the process. I must learn to carefully analyze my actions (something which requires a great deal of skill and understanding of which I have little at present); but this is the only way I will learn to think before I act, to respond to my perceptions, and to be clear about my purpose.

A third student wrote her summary in two stages, the first when utterly discouraged, and the second, after she had worked through her discouragement and gained insight that enabled her to see her strengths and her potentialities in clearer perspective.

If a month ago someone had said to me: 'Would you please go up to the maternity unit and give them a hand up there, they're very short of help today,' I don't think I would have batted an eye. I would perhaps have had a small degree of apprehension because I did not know the physical set-up on that ward, but I certainly would have felt quite confident in my ability to give nursing care to a half-dozen new mothers and their babies. . . . But this week, the thought of meeting face-to-face just *one* mother has struck panic in me: a fright bordering on nightmare. Why? Why is it that I am so afraid?

Did I, all of a sudden, over night, turn from a 'good' nurse into a 'bad' one? Or have I ever been a 'good' nurse? Or for that matter, have I ever defined for myself what a good nurse and what a bad nurse is, and on what bases had I evaluated myself and my work anyway? Have I ever really known what I was doing and why? Is this fear of contact with patients really so sudden or have I always had it, and been unable to admit it to myself?

The snowball of doubts and fears has started rolling and it is gathering speed and size. I feel as if my comfortable little world has been knocked right out from under me, and I am very much afraid for myself. One thing I know. I cannot possibly be of any use to a patient when I am so paralyzed with self-concern. . . . I need help.

The following day the student added this to her summary:

As you can see, last night I went to bed with a terrible feeling of despair. I could not go to sleep for a long time; I kept thinking. This morning I read what I had written last night—matters seemed still as bad yet somehow not as hopeless. The morning was so beautiful!. . . I went out for a walk. I walked for three hours and, when I returned, exhausted and refreshed, I sat down to write what I had come up with during my long walk.

So I am afraid to face a patient. But I have admitted it to myself! I have gone farther than that. I have admitted it to you, and what's more, for the first time in my life I have had the guts to put it down on paper—in black and white. Why, that's hope in itself!

So now that I have admitted it . . . I am going to look at my fear. And I'll start by asking myself what is it that I'm afraid of. The answer comes as a hard blow. My fear is not for the patient—that I may do her damage by failing to provide her with what she needs. My fear is a self-centered one. I am afraid of failure. I am afraid that I may prove myself to be inadequate in my own eyes, in the eyes of my classmates and in your eyes.

But this is my consolation. When I define and accept the purpose of my being with patients, the purpose will guide my steps. The purpose will provide a means to measure my failure and to examine it. Perhaps the realization of my purpose will free me from self-concern enough to make me useful to my patients. Examined, measured and accepted, failure may become a tool for learning.

If I can learn to expect and accept the expectation of failure without fear, I may be freed enough from self-concern to be able to think and act in terms of my purpose when I finally define and accept it.

Students in schools of nursing—be they basic or graduate schools—are mature individuals. They are, for the most part, members of today's group of young people who have been described by Chris Argyris as desiring "an education that is relevant for twentieth-century problems; an education that will help them to fulfill their trust and responsibility for the makeup of this society.

Many of the students are much more sophisticated than their predecessors. . . . Students are acquiring knowledge earlier and in greater quantities than ever before. They know more about the world and its problems. They are exposed to analysis, the world of thought, earlier and more intensively than ever before.

Many are . . . professionals. They value competence more than any attribute. They have come to educate themselves, to obtain knowledge so that they can do something with this knowledge. For the most part, they are a nononsense generation who expect others and themselves to practice what they preach. . . . They want to be confronted with the problems of our society.

The maturity and the dedication of the present student generation have been underestimated and misunderstood by the universities. Many students are ready for education that integrates thought with action, inquiry with policy. The absence of such education is a basic source of student discontent.*

Such assessment of students' aspirations, capabilities and interests suggests that it may be important for the clinical instructor to examine the thoughts she may hold about her students—how she regards them, and what assumptions she has made about them and on what she bases her assumptions. Her

---
* Chris Argyris, "Some Consequences of Separating Thought From Action," *Ventures*, Spring 1968, p. 69.

assumptions determine, in large measure, her attitude toward her students and guide her in her effort to develop, with each student, an authentic relationship that is conducive to learning. Consequently, the instructor may find it important to sort out her assumptions, list them, determine their sources and significance, and let them serve her in her work with students.

The following list of assumptions is presented in the hope that it will stimulate other instructors to make their own assumptions explicit and then use them as guides in the development of the kind of relationships they hope to establish with their students.

Assumption 1. The student is a potentially capable individual. Since students are human beings, they are endowed with facilities for functioning that enable them to think, reason, feel, sense, perceive and act. They also have reached an age of relative maturity. The minimum age for admission to basic schools of nursing is generally 18, but many students, especially those in university schools—graduate and undergraduate—are considerably older and have had a variety of maturing life experiences. Furthermore, students are admitted to schools of nursing only if they have met specific, and usually rigid, requirements relating to academic preparation and achievement, health, professional competence (when application is to a graduate school) and personal attributes and attitudes. Consequently, they are believed to be well able to grasp the content of the school's program and to participate competently in its activities.

Assumption 2. Whatever the student does represents her best judgment at the moment of doing it. This assumption is founded on the belief that the judgment on which a student bases her action at any given moment, derives from the clarity with which she views the situation she is experiencing at the instant that action is imminent; and from the availability to her, at that same moment, of resources she may have for dealing with the situation. Such resources include knowledge, understanding, motivation, strength, energy and essential equipment. The student's view and the availability of her resources are unique to her at that particular moment and are reflected in the action she takes. The judgment and resultant action of another person in the same situation might be quite different because he will view the situation differently and a different set of resources will be available to him. Likewise, when looking back on the situation at a later time, the student might view it in broader perspective and her resources might be more clearly recognizable and, consequently more available to her than they were at the moment of actually experiencing the situation. In retrospect, therefore, her judgment of what to do might be different and suggest a different kind of action. Thus, the student's perception and the accessibility to her of her resources are key factors in determining the action she takes at any given moment, and need to be recognized and given consideration in any appraisal of the action that the instructor might make.

Assumption 3. The student usually applies for admission to a school because she wants to participate in the kind of program she thinks the school is offering. A student usually selects, of her own volition, the school to which she applied. She generally makes her selection because, among other factors, she is impressed by the kind of program she thinks the school offers. Her assumptions about the program are based on what she may have read in the school catalogue or what she may have heard about it. If a discrepancy exists between the student's assumption and the actuality, she may develop unrealistic expectations. This can cause disillusionment and frustration that may seriously interfere with the student's ability to learn. Consequently, should the instructor suspect that such a problem is plaguing the student, she may want to try to find out what the student's expectations were before she entered the program and try to reconcile any discrepancy between these expectations and the actualities that exist.

Assumption 4. The student will both seek and accept help from the instructor if she believes that the instructor is accepting of her. The student tends to view the instructor as a person who wields power and authority. She knows that the instructor evaluates her work and assigns to it a grade that affects the student's standing in the school and her eligibility for promotion or graduation. At the same time, she is apt to regard the instructor as knowledgeable and competent and to believe that she has potential for giving the kind of help the student may need. Hence, she may fear the instructor; but on the other hand, she may feel she needs her. Such conflict militates against the student's ability to seek help easily.

To some students, this conflict presents no particular problem. They realize that they are in school to learn; that if they knew all the answers they would not have come; and they trust the instructor. Consequently, they participate enthusiastically in class, share their ideas and questions and expose their knowledge and actions willingly for critical analysis and for the insights they may gain from doing so, and they seek help when they recognize their need for it.

To other students, however, the conflict does present a problem. Some of them appear to try to ignore it. They may participate actively in class but only in a general way. They tend to be reluctant to reveal their uncertainties or to expose their knowledge and actions, and they neither seek the instructor's help nor show interest in her assessment of their progress. The instructor may be able to break down their defenses and reach them, but it may take her a long time to do so. Individual conferences may be helpful in giving her opportunity to encourage the student and to take the initiative in presenting her own impressions or concerns regarding problems she thinks the student may be experiencing. She also may be able to break down the student's defenses through candid and specific responses to her summaries of thinking.

Still other students to whom the conflict presents a problem try to take steps to resolve it. To them, the instructor is definitely suspect and they seem to feel that they must determine, either by questioning her directly or by subjecting her to a process of testing, whether they can admit to her that they need her help. One student, for example, asked the instructor every week over a period of two months, how the instructor was evaluating her work; another expressed her belief that the instructor regarded her as incapable of learning; still another frankly stated her distrust. Further examples are the student who took issue with the instructor over the way the instructor conducted a class, and the student who, when told by the instructor that she as well as the others in her group, could choose how each would like to be oriented to the clinical area, responded that she would like to sit in a wheelchair and observe what went on on the floor. All of these students, in one way or another, tried to put the instructor "on the spot." By doing so, however, they gave her opportunity to assure them of her acceptance of them, an assurance they apparently needed in order to be able to seek and accept her help.

Assumption 5. The older a student is, the more difficult it may be for her to accept herself as a learner. The older student, the one who is past the age of adolescence and who, before entering the school of nursing, has had a number of years of experience in such activities as teaching, business, nursing (if she is a graduate student), travelling or in being wife and mother, often has difficulty adjusting to her new role of student. It may not be easy for her to regulate her life to the exigencies of classes, schedules and assignments. She may be disturbed by her need to alter her ways of thinking and functioning that years of experience have fashioned into fairly firmly fixed patterns. Although she may apply herself diligently to her studies and be meticulous and prompt in carrying out her responsibilities, she tends to cover her uncertainties and anxieties with a manner that seems aggressive, self-protective or hypersensitive. She may, for example, try to dominate class discussion by challenging, almost with an inquisitor's zeal, statements the instructor or a classmate might make. She may recount at length and in great detail, personal experiences she has had, or introduce extraneous topics, thus digressing from the subject under consideration. Another such student may seldom express an opinion of her own, but readily quote those of others; or, she may ask minute directions before undertaking any activity and indicate concern lest she not do it "exactly right;" she may even burst into tears if asked to justify an action. Should the instructor be younger than the student (a situation that not infrequently occurs, especially in graduate school), the student may try to avoid the instructor, asking almost anyone rather than her, for information or help. She may be hypercritical of everything the instructor may do or say, or she may act resentful, sarcastic or even condescending when the instructor calls on her in class, gives her an assignment, makes a suggestion or offers help. Such behaviors, when manifested by an older student (regardless of what the age differential between her and the instructor may be) are usually indicative of her extreme discomfort in her student role and call for the instructor's understanding, tolerance and restraint. Such attitudes and actions of the student actually defeat her purpose in coming to the school and may hamper her ability to learn. The instructor may be able to help the student to overcome her block by trying, in a supportive way, to get her to recognize the inconsistencies she is presenting. This may require: 1) frequent assurance by the instructor that she believes the student has potential for capable functioning; 2) candid responses to the student's challenges; 3) requests that the student particularize when she generalizes, or that she express *her* opinions or reactions rather than those of others; 4) initiative in offering help when the instructor thinks the student may need it; and 5) commendation for any act well done. In addition, the instructor who is younger than the student may buoy up her own spirits by reminding herself that, although the student may be the more experienced of the two in many aspects of life, she, the instructor, is more knowledgeable and experienced than the student in the content and conduct of *this* program and, consequently, has much that is valuable to offer the student.

Besides the assumptions about student motivation and qualities described in the foregoing paragraphs, the instructor may also find it useful to add to the list some assumptions that are suggestive of student needs, including:

Assumption 6. The student needs encouragement, help and opportunity to make best use of the facilities for functioning with which she is endowed. Every student is able to sense, think, speak and act. She is endowed with facilities that make such abilities possible; that is, she has sensory organs, a mind, nervous and motor systems. As a result, she often makes excellent observations, discerns inconsistencies, and has ideas about what might help a patient in need, but then, when in the clinical area, ignores them in the actions she takes.

One student, for example, after caring for a patient who had had an abdominal operation three days earlier, expressed her frustration to her instructor because the patient continued to complain of backache, in spite of all the measures the student had used to try to ease it. She said the patient had asked for a supportive binder but that, instead of trying to get one for her, she had rubbed her back, helped her change her position, adjusted pillows and placed an extra one under her knees.

"Those are all good measures," the instructor commended her, but added, "What about the binder?"

"Oh," the student replied, "I think they're not allowed, so I didn't even try to get one."

"Did you ask any one if your patient might have one?" the instructor inquired.

"No-o-o" the student said, somewhat wonderingly.

"Why don't you ask the doctor?" the instructor suggested. "He's right over there."

The student acted on this suggestion and then, smiling broadly, told the instructor that the doctor had raised no objections; in fact, he thought using the binder a good idea.

Another student indicated her concern, in conference, because a young pregnant woman for whom she had cared, was in the hospital for the third time in three weeks because of excessive weight gain.

"She's a college graduate," the student said, "she knows what to eat and what to avoid, and she says she could have the same kind of food at home as she has here. But she doesn't stick to her diet when she's home. It doesn't make sense."

"Nice observation," the instructor commented. "What did you do about it?"

"Well, I discussed her diet with her," the student answered, "and the importance of staying with it during these last few weeks of her pregnancy. I suggested substitutions that she could make for salt, for instance, and ways of cooking foods to make them more palatable. She seemed to understand, and I hope she'll be able to stick to her diet this time!"

"I hope she can too," the instructor concurred," but isn't that wishful thinking?"

The student looked surprised, and so the instructor continued, "What makes you think she'll stay with her diet any better when she gets home than she did before?"

"I think I went into greater detail with her," the student explained, a bit defensively. "She could tell me exactly what she had been eating at home, and I think I helped her to realize why it was important for her, and the baby, that she follow the diet that had been prescribed."

"Did you try to find out why she hadn't been able to in the past?" the instructor asked.

"No, not especially," the student replied. "She'd said before that she doesn't like unsalted food and doesn't care for what they serve in the hospital."

"But what about the inconsistency you said you had noted? Remember? You said it didn't make sense to you that this educated young woman, couldn't stick to her diet when she was at home. That seems strange to me too. Maybe there is something in her home situation that makes adherence to diet impossible for her. Maybe she's evidencing resistance to having the baby—maybe—oh, there are all kinds of reasons that might be at the root of her problem."

"That's true," the student said, thoughtfully.

"You made such excellent observations, you were sensitive to the inconsistencies in them and were baffled by them. I wonder, why you didn't respect them and act on them?"

"I don't know," replied the student. "I guess I was just so concerned about the diet and what she could do about it, I never thought to find out why she hadn't been able to follow it at home." Then she added wryly, "As a matter of fact, I never even tried to find out whether she needed to know all that I did tell her!"

All too frequently, students who want to help their patients and go to great lengths to try to do so, fail to get the kind of results from their efforts that they hoped to get. Their failure, as in the incidents just described, may be due to lack of respect for their facilities for functioning and to unvalidated assumptions that interfere with their following through on good ideas they may have. However, when they are helped to recognize not only how and why they ignored their perceptions, reactions and ideas, but also how they might have used them to obtain desired results, they have the basis for developing insights that can make their future nursing actions more meaningful and rewarding.

Assumption 7. The student needs to feel secure in her ability to function before she is able to give effective, comprehensive care to patients. Dexterity, deftness, efficiency—these are qualities frequently exhibited by nurses and aspired to by students. When observing a nurse at work, for instance, a student may marvel at her skilled use of hands, the swiftness with which she can set up a table with sterile instruments, bowls and sponges for surgical use, or the sureness with which she gently turns a patient who is heavy, helpless and in pain. She yearns to display such competencies herself, for she, and others too, regard them as the hallmarks of a nurse. Consequently, a student may anticipate her first clinical experience with trepidation and anxiety, not so much for fear that she will harm the patient as for fear that she may seem clumsy, stupid or inept to other nurses, doctors or even to her instructor. Such anxiety can build up and defeat her at every turn in the clinical area when she tries to carry out her assignment for patient care. Until she feels reasonably secure in her ability to function according to what she expects of herself and what she thinks others expect of her, clinical experience may be traumatic to a serious degree. Her instructor's presence in the area, although intended to be reassuring, often aggravates the student's fear. But if the student has been helped to prepare herself in advance for what she will be expected to do and how to do it, she may be able to look forward to her experience in the clinical area with eager anticipation and peace of mind. Such preparation might include: 1) becoming familiar with the physical layout of the area; 2) being able to practice various procedures that often need to be carried out; 3) having opportunity to try out or manipulate special pieces of equipment; and 4) being assured that the instructor will be there to help should she be needed. To become prepared, the student may require more time than is usually allotted to orientation of a student for a clinical experience, or the goal of the usual orientation may need to be refocused. In any case, if provision is made for meeting the student's need to feel secure, the value to her of the clinical experience may be greatly enhanced.

Assumption 8. The student needs opportunity to apply in practice, concepts she has learned. The fact that a student indicates that she understands a concept, does not necessarily mean that she is able to apply it. The gap that seems to exist between avowed mental grasp and implementation can best be bridged through clinical practice that is instructor-supported and directed toward the student's learning.

In one class discussion, for example, the students' comments, questions and responses showed that they recognized the importance of identifying a patient's need for help before giving help that they might think is needed. Yet, the following day, when the instructor saw a student standing at the desk flipping the pages of a chart and asked her what she was looking for, the student's reply was, "Mrs. Black says her stomach hurts and I thought I'd see if she has a p.r.n. order for medication."

The instructor was puzzled. What do you mean by 'her stomach hurts'? Can you be more specific?"

"Well, no, not really," the student answered. "She looks as though she is in pain and she was rubbing her lower abdomen and said it hurt."

"Uh-huh," the instructor nodded in understanding, "Those are all pretty good signs that something's bothering her, but what makes you think that pain medication will help her? Might she possibly need a bed pan, or a suppository, or even a doctor?"

The student grimaced as the instructor spoke, and then burst out, as though disgusted with herself, "I never tried to find out what she really might need! I didn't look at her abdomen or feel it, and didn't even ask her anything about her pain. I was just going to go ahead and try to relieve it!"

"Your intention was good," the instructor smiled, "but that's not the best way to go about trying to meet a patient's need for help."

"It certainly is not!" the student declared emphatically. "I'll go back and see what I can find out."

This incident illustrates how classroom learning of concepts requires reinforcement in practice. The student's desire to be helpful to her patient was unquestioned. The true meaning of the concept of helping escaped her, however, until she discovered herself in the act of violating it. Unless there is opportunity for the student to apply nursing concepts in practice, learning them in the classroom can become merely an academic exercise.

Assumption 9. The student needs to know how the instructor views her progress in the course she is taking. Students need and want to know how the instructor is evaluating their progress and the quality of their work as the course progresses. Grades are important to them and probably have been, ever since childhood when rewards and penalties often were associated with the report cards they brought home. Grades can also be regarded as an instructor's secret weapon that she can use with deadly aim. Accounts of students "flunking out" of school without previous warning are on record and every student knows that the possibility exists that that might happen to her.

Students manifest their anxiety about their progress in a variety of ways. One may ask directly how the instructor thinks she is progressing. Another may withdraw when in the instructor's presence for fear that whatever she may say or do will be held against her. Still another may be reluctant to ask the instructor outright how she is doing, but confide to someone close to the instructor, possibly an assistant, that she would like to know just where she stands, in the instructor's eyes. Or, a student may casually introduce the subject of evaluation into a conference discussion and eagerly respond to the instructor's offer to discuss the progress she thinks the student has made.

A student's anxiety about her instructor's view of her progress may be relieved, to a large degree, if the quality of her work is discussed with her at stated intervals throughout the year. Her concern is well-founded, for she knows that her promotion and even her eligibility for graduation are dependent, to a considerable extent, on her grades. She needs to know where she stands before it is too late for her to do something about it, should her work seem less than satisfactory; and she may need assurance, too, that her instructor believes that she can improve the quality of her work.

Ideally, one may say that a student's concern should be to meet her own standards of excellence rather than those of her instructor. Realistically, however, the current educational system places a premium on instructor-given grades, and this precludes such a switch in attitude.

Assumption 10. The student needs opportunity to express her feelings frankly to her instructor. Learning experiences that are directed toward effecting change in thinking, attitude and ways of doing may be stimulating and exciting for the student, particularly in a practice discipline. They can also be baffling, threatening and disturbing. Opportunities to think clearly about her philosophy and purpose and try to be true to them in what she does; to serve patients suffering from all kinds of ailments and afflictions yet respond to them with objectivity, warmth and understanding; and to associate with men and women whose interests are humanitarian and to feel the thrill of becoming one of them are all challenging experiences, especially when they are coupled with the realization that in her hands may rest, at any time, the life and welfare of a human being.

Students vary in the way they respond to each day's challenges. Some identify with every patient's illness and discover that they, too, have symptoms similar to those their patients have displayed. Some feel elated when a concept becomes clear to them and reveals entirely new ways of functioning. Some feel devastated when they realize that their actions in the past were based mostly on unvalidated assumptions and that what is past is past and cannot be corrected now.

Often students share their fears, questions, pleasures and anxieties with their classmates and, as a rule, they seem also to welcome the opportunity to discuss them, individually and confidentially, with their instructor. They may not take the initiative in making appointments to talk with her, but will "drop in" when they see her office door open. If the instructor sets up a schedule of when she will be available and assigns a special time for each student, the students will usually appear at the appointed time and will have in mind questions and problems they would like to discuss. Sometimes a student finds it easier to write what is on her mind than to say it in conference. For her, a device such as a summary of thinking may prove useful, especially if she knows that the instructor will respect the personal nature of her comments and that she can count on a written personal reply.

• • • • • • • • • • •

The Framework

The framework of a clinical teaching program is made up of a complex of factors which, though formless and intangible in their entirety, have, nevertheless, potential for limiting or expanding the scope of the instructor's ability to function at any given time. It derives from elements and circumstances, imagined or real, that are present or are introduced into every teaching situation and which, by their existence, shape the course of events. In addition, they influence not only the ease with which the instructor is able to carry out her plans, but also the facility with which the student is able to learn. Such factors and circumstances may be the community, school, hospital, classroom or clinical area, with all of their appurtenances. They may be people actually present in a situation, or whose presence is anticipated, and those who may arrive unexpectedly or whose memory may pervade the instructor's—or the student's—consciousness. They also may be atmospheric conditions, time of day and happenings that by their occurrence may promote, complicate, alter, impair or impede the carrying out of the instructor's plans.

The following incidents are suggestive of the variety of ways in which the framework may manifest itself and influence the course of events.

1. Just as the instructor was about to go to the clinical area for a morning's experience there with her students, she met the director of nurses who stopped her to express appreciation for the fine work that two of the students

had done in caring for a particularly frightened cardiac patient, and that the supervisor had told her about. As the director talked, the instructor felt a warm glow of pride and pleasure suffuse her; in fact, she felt as though "her day had been made!" Subsequently, she entered upon the morning's activities with renewed zest. Furthermore, she let the students know how pleased she was to be given such a fine report about their work, thus giving their morale a boost that they, in turn, reflected in their enthusiastic responsiveness throughout the morning.

In this incident, the framework, epitomized by the director of nurses and her comments of appreciation, inspired the instructor and, indirectly, the students to go "beyond the call of duty" in carrying out her plans and their assignments.

2. The instructor had arranged for the showing of a special film as an introduction to her class on The Hospitalized Patient and His Need for Help. A thunderstorm had been threatening and, just as the students assembled, it broke loose. Then the electric power failed. Not only could the film not be shown, but the room was plunged into darkness and this necessitated moving the entire class to another area as well as reorganizing its conduct.

Thus, the thunderstorm, a dominant part of the situation's framework, effectively blocked the instructor in her effort to carry out her plans.

3. In the course of a morning's experience with her students, a particular instructor was called to the telephone. The long distance call was from her sister asking her to come home because their father was desperately ill. This unexpected news and request had a shattering effect on the instructor. Questions raced through her mind. How long might her father live? What time could she catch a plane? How would her mother manage without him? Could she get to the bank in time to cash a check? Would her father be alive when she got home? Who would take over her class schedule while she was

gone? So much of her mind was taken up with her personal problems that she could apply only a small portion of it to her students' needs for help. Although present with them in the clinical area, she was available to them to only a limited extent. She was well aware of her inadequacy but felt unable to cope with it. Consequently, she dismissed the students as soon as they had completed their assignments and cancelled the usual post-experience conference.

In this incident, the framework, in the semblance of the sister's message and the chain of thoughts it loosed, had an inhibiting effect on the instructor and obstructed her efforts to implement her plans.

4. When the instructor arrived on the clinical unit with her students, she found it in a state of confusion. Partially filled food carts stood in the corridors. Breakfast trays with soiled dishes and uneaten food sat on bedside tables or on chairs. Patients looked disheveled and glum. Linen shelves were empty. Charts were in use by doctors making rounds. An orderly was sweeping. Workmen were repairing the ceiling. The nurse in charge, substituting for the head nurse who was on vacation, was trying to give assignments to the nursing staff and at the same time to bring some order out of the chaos. The instructor had planned for her students to be in the clinical area three hours that particular morning. Instead of devoting that block of time to a productive experience with patients, however, both she and the students spent a good half of it on such preliminary tasks as removing breakfast trays, searching for linen, waiting for charts to be released by the doctors, hunting for the nurse in charge to consult her about some "order" or a need a patient had expressed, or finding an orderly and trying to cajole him into mopping a section of the floor around a patient's bed where spilled coffee had formed a large, unsightly slippery spot.

The framework of this incident, represented by the clinical unit's state of disarray and confusion, prevented the instructor from carrying out her plans and also interfered with the students' learning experience. Thus, the framework, although amorphous and indefinable as a whole, is, nevertheless, as much a part of the teaching situation as are the instructor and the students. It is a multi-segmented aspect of the realities and, because it inevitably exerts a powerful influence on the instructor's course of action as well as on the students' ability to learn, it is a force to be reckoned with deliberately.

What matters particularly about the framework is not so much the fact of its pervasive presence as the use the instructor makes of it in her teaching program. It has tremendous potential for influencing learning. When the instructor realizes this, respects the framework and uses it adroitly, it can contribute significantly to the broadening of the students' perspectives, the enhancement of their objectivity, the clarification of their purposes, and to the gaining of insights that will contribute meaningfully to their competence in nursing. The following incidents illustrate this point.

1. In a post-experience conference, a student voiced her indignation over having been asked by the head nurse to take a patient in a wheelchair to the x-ray department on another floor.

"I went," the student said, "but I was churning all the way. Taking a patient to x-ray is not part of my responsibility, but that's what always happens! Just because we're students and handy, nurses on the floor ask us to do things the orderly or maid should be doing—only they're not always easy to find!"

As she spoke, some of the students sitting around the table looked thoughtful; others nodded their heads in agreement.

The instructor concurred that at times students are asked to do things that seem extraneous to their reason for being in the area, and expressed understanding of the student's reactions. She also commended her for expressing her feelings frankly in the conference. She pointed out however, that the situation was a realistic one and that the students could expect to be faced with similar ones again. Therefore, she indicated, the question is not so much how to prevent a staff member from making such a request of a student, but rather, how can the student deal with it constructively.

The ensuing discussion was lively. It brought out that: 1) the student had complied with the request to take the patient to the x-ray department without raising any question or making any comment about her reaction to the head nurse at the time; 2) the student did not know what circumstances had caused the head nurse to ask her, rather than the orderly, to do this assignment; 3) the student was not involved in some activity that could not be readily interrupted at the time the request was made; and 4) a patient often feels more secure when being taken to some other part of the hospital if accompanied by a nurse who is concerned about her welfare and who would know what to do should something untoward occur.

The students indicated further their recognition that: a) for emergent or unusual reasons, it may be legitimate for the head nurse to ask a student or a nurse to carry out some non-nursing function, and for the student or the nurse to do so; but when such requests become habitual, steps to stop them may need to be taken; b) a student, especially when she is burning with indignation, may have responsibility—in the interest of her relationship with the patient and the head nurse and of her own peace of mind—to find out how the head nurse happened to ask the student rather than some one like the orderly, to take the patient to x-ray; but that 3) the student must use her judgment about a) whether to try to find this out at the time or afterwards, and b) how to go about trying to find this out; and 4) if the student is uncertain about how to approach the head nurse with her question, she should try to discuss the problem with her instructor in an effort to find a satisfactory solution.

The instructor thus tried to have the students view the framework—in this incident, the head nurse and her request—in broader perspective than the one in which the student initially saw it, and to gain from it insights that would help them cope constructively with such situations in the future.

2. Three students, huddled together in the utility room on the hospital's medical unit, were carrying on an animated dis-

cussion. As the instructor approached them, she heard one of them say:

"Well, if I were in charge of this floor, you sure wouldn't see such dirt and disorder in the patients' rooms!"

"What's going on here?" the instructor asked. "Sounds like a major gripe session!"

The students looked embarrassed. Then one of them said: "Yes, that's exactly what we're having. Peggy was just telling us. . . ."

Before she could finish her sentence, the student named Peggy burst out, "You should see the dirt in that room I was in! And the mess! Big rolls of dust and lint under the beds. Soot on the window sills. And I bet those bedside tables haven't been cleaned in months!"

"Must be awful," the instructor agreed. "But what are you planning to do about it?"

The students looked surprised and one of them asked, "We? Why, what can—should—*we* do about it?"

"That's a good question," the instructor responded. "But, why were you all talking together? Were you trying to figure out something to do about it?"

"No," Peggy answered. "We were just comparing notes, and I guess giving vent to our disgust or something!"

"That's fair enough," the instructor said. "It's a good idea, sometimes, to let off steam when you're boiling inside, but that doesn't particularly help the situation, or does it?"

"Well, no, not really," another student answered. "I guess maybe we're being too critical."

"Oh, I doubt that," the instructor responded. "It shows that you have some pretty high standards and are concerned because what you have observed on the unit falls far short of them."

"Yes," the student agreed, "I guess that's true."

"It's fine to be aware of what seems to be wrong and to give expression to your distress about it," the instructor continued. "If you leave it at that, though, you are just registering your dismay, and any one can do that!"

"What would you want us to do?" the third student asked, and then she added, somewhat sarcastically, "Clean up the place?"

"That's one thing you could do, I guess," the instructor responded, "but that might not have a lasting effect."

"No," Peggy agreed with a shrug. "Next week it would probably be just as bad as ever."

"It sounds to me as though you're being critical without really knowing what all is involved," the instructor countered.

"What do you mean?" Peggy asked.

"I'm just expressing the thought that permanently keeping the room clean may be more complicated than it might seem to be, at first glance."

The students listened questioningly, and the instructor continued, "What you are really saying, you know, is that something needs to be changed. Specifically, the room needs to be clean and orderly rather than dirty and disorderly. That's an important recognition. But then you also need to identify exactly what changes are needed. And that gets a little more complicated. Can you, for instance, suggest what they might be?"

"Oh yes," Peggy was quick to answer. "The floor should be swept every day instead of only occasionally. It should be mopped or waxed at least once a week instead of—I don't know how often it's done now."

"Not very often, I bet!" one of the other students injected.

Then Peggy continued, "Bedside tables should be inspected. I think they never are now. They should be thoroughly scrubbed, too, when a patient is discharged and I'm sure that isn't current practice!"

As Peggy paused, the instructor said, "That's a good list to start with. The changes you suggest seem reasonable. But now, how would you bring those changes about?"

"Hmmm," Peggy mused, "if I were the head nurse, I think I'd assign the job of daily sweeping to the orderly, for one thing, and then...."

"Wait a minute," the instructor interjected. "Maybe you have forgotten, or don't realize, that the head nurse in this hospital has no authority over the orderly and does not give him his assignments. He is on the housekeeping staff, and that is under the jurisdiction of hospital administration."

"Oh," Peggy exclaimed, somewhat taken aback. "Then you mean the head nurse isn't really responsible for the condition of the floor and bedside tables in patients' rooms?"

"Only indirectly," the instructor said, "and partially."

"Well," Peggy said, "that does make a difference. Then would I have to talk to someone in the administrative department, like the unit manager or housekeeper, and persuade him to arrange for an orderly to sweep daily?"

"Oh, and then you might have to follow up that talk," one of the other students remarked, "to make sure the assignment had been given to the orderly!"

"But then," Peggy asked wonderingly, "would I have to go through administration every time I wanted the orderly to do something?"

"That's something you'd have to find out from the administrator," the instructor answered.

"Gee, it's more complicated than I thought," Peggy exclaimed. "I guess we had better think about what all's involved in making changes, before sounding off about what's wrong!"

The instructor tried, throughout this discussion, to have the students view the framework, i.e., the disorderly room, objectively rather than merely emotionally, and to recognize their responsibility to follow their observation that something needed to be done about it with suggestions as to what specifically should be done and how, realistically, to bring about the desired changes.

3. The instructor was at Mrs. Smith's bedside with a student who had consulted her about a breast feeding problem Mrs. Smith seemed to be having. The mother had difficulty fitting her nipple as well as the areola into the baby's little mouth, but finally, with assistance, succeeded. The baby was just starting to nurse well, when the nursery nurse suddenly appeared, walked to the bed and, with arms extended as if to take the baby, said, "Dr. Johnson wants to examine the baby, so I've come to get her."

Mrs. Smith looked up and tensed. The student looked startled, and the instructor, startled too, said, "Wait a minute. The baby has just latched on and started to nurse well." Then, looking first at the mother and then at the student, added, "I think Mrs. Smith would rather not interrupt the baby's feeding right now."

The mother nodded, relaxed visibly, and turned her attention back to the baby.

The nursery nurse dropped her arms to her sides, backed up a bit, and hesitatingly said, "But Dr. Johnson asked me to bring him the baby."

"I know," the instructor replied understandingly, "but he probably didn't realize that the baby had just started to nurse well—quite an achievement, too, for she had difficulty getting hold of the nipple." Then, catching the student's eye and noting her approving and relieved look, continued, "Do please tell Dr. Johnson how it is," and, glancing again at the student, added, "Miss Trevor will bring the baby to the nursery for him to examine in about twenty minutes. O.K.?"

The student nodded her agreement, and the nursery nurse, looking from one to the other, said in a low voice as though to herself, "I'll tell him and see how he takes it!"

"Thanks," said the instructor to the nursery nurse who withdrew, shaking her head as though unconvinced that the pediatrician would agree to postponement of his intended examination of the baby.

Later that morning, after the baby had successfully nursed and had been examined, the instructor was able to discuss this particular incident with the student. They talked about the instructor's reason for taking over the student's function when the nursery nurse arrived, and about the nurse's need to be clear about her purpose in nursing, especially when some element in the framework (in this case the nursery nurse and, indirectly, the pediatrician) intrudes in order to take care of a need of its own, regardless of the importance of what the nurse and patient might be doing. The discussion brought out, too, that it was important for the nurse to respect the need presented by the so-called "framework," and to suggest how it might be met in a mutually acceptable way. Following their discussion and prior to leaving the clinical area, the instructor and the student stopped at the nursery to thank the nurse for her response and to tell her how much it seemed to mean to the mother to be able to nurse her baby without interruption.

4. A student, flushed and frowning, sought the clinical instructor and, on finding her, voiced her indignation over the head nurse's seeming indifference to her wish to help a mother, Mrs. Tompkins, care for her baby.

"She's going home tomorrow," the student explained earnestly. "This is her first baby and she's never even so much as changed a baby's diaper. And she's scared!"

"Would she like you to show her how?" the instructor asked.

"Oh, yes," the student replied emphatically. "She asked me to show her how to dress and undress the baby and to let her try doing it herself before she goes home. She said she has no one there to help her—her husband has had no experience either—but when I asked Miss Gray, she said there's no time now to do that."

"So," the instructor smiled as she asked, "what's your suggestion."

"Well," the student hesitatingly answered, "I wondered if maybe you'd talk to the head nurse?"

"I suppose I could, but let's talk about it first and see if that's really what you'd like me to do." The student indicated her agreement, and so the instructor continued, "Tell me, if you can, just what you said to Miss Gray, what she said to you and then what you did."

"Well," the student recalled, "first of all, when Mrs. Tompkins told me how concerned she was, I told her I'd try to get her baby from the nursery and hold a practice session with her. I thought it would be all right to do that if I put on a gown and pulled the screen curtain around us just as we do when a mother nurses her baby. I had finished my assignment, too, so I had the time to give to Mrs. Tompkins. Then I went to find Miss Gray. She was standing by the desk, talking to the ward secretary. I interrupted them, excusing myself first, of course, and asked if it would be all right for me to give Mrs. Tompkins a baby care demonstration because she hadn't had one. And then Miss Gray told me, as I said before, 'There's no time to do that now!' So," the student shrugged her shoulders, "I don't know just what to do. Mrs. Tompkins needs that demonstration and experience, and I'd like to give it to her."

"You are kind of on the spot," the instructor mused aloud. "Do you think Miss Gray realizes how much Mrs. Tompkins would like to have that practice?"

"Oh, sure she does," the student was quick to answer. "Why, I told her she'd never had a demonstration."

"Yes," the instructor said, "but you know, lots of mothers haven't had one. When you told me about the problem though, you made me think that you were really very concerned about Mrs. Tompkins' inexperience and anxiety, and that you had an idea about how you might help her. Do you think you got that thought over to Miss Gray?"

"Well," the student was thoughtful as she answered, "I guess I just assumed she'd know. No, I merely asked to give Mrs. Tompkins a demonstration because she hadn't had one. I probably should have told her why. But," she added defensively, "even if I had, she'd probably have said 'No'."

"That's a pretty big assumption," the instructor said. "Do you really think Miss Gray would let Mrs. Tompkins go home without a demonstration if she knew how badly she wanted one? That's not the way she's impressed me. In fact, I've known her to do many thoughtful, helpful things for mothers."

"Actually, I have, too," the student conceded, "but she certainly wasn't interested when I spoke to her."

"No," the instructor agreed, "but it sounds to me as though you really hadn't gotten your message across."

The student smiled sheepishly, then asked, "What'll I do?"

"Could you ask Miss Gray again, do you think?"

"And be more explicit?"

"Yes," the instructor replied, "but mostly, try to let Miss Gray know how much you care and why."

"I guess I could," the student said. "But how'll I start? I hate to interrupt her again. And she was very definite when she said 'No'."

"Tell her just the way it is," the instructor suggested. "Let her know you hate to interrupt her again, but that you are concerned and think perhaps you didn't fully explain why it seems so important to you to give Mrs. Tompkins an opportunity to dress and undress the baby before she goes home."

"Yes," the student agreed, "I could say that, and if she says 'There's no time to do it now' again, I could suggest doing it at a later time."

"Good idea," the instructor commented. "But rather than your suggesting a later time, what would you think of asking Miss Gray to suggest a more convenient time and indicating that you'd be glad to come any time she might suggest, either today or tomorrow morning, provided of course, that you do have the time."

"Yes, I have the time," the student responded. "I'll try, and I'll let you know what happens."

"Good!" the instructor exclaimed. "I'll be eager to hear."

Later in the afternoon, a radiant student greeted the instructor and told her the head nurse had been very understanding when the student had spoken to her again. Miss Gray had even suggested that the student give the demonstration in the early evening, during visiting hours, when perhaps the husband would be there too. She also had offered the student use of a side room where the demonstration might be held.

The instructor, of course, expressed her pleasure that the student had succeeded in gaining the head nurse's consent, and wished her well in her plan for the evening. She had a feeling of satisfaction, too, for she believed that the student had gained some useful insights from this experience that would help her in the future to meet similar resistance within the framework and to gain permission to do something that a patient might desire, and which she, as the nurse, might think essential and want very much to do.

As suggested by these four stories, the framework can impinge in innumerable ways on the clinical instructor's activities and plans. It presents a major challenge to her as well as to the student. It is dynamic, often unpredictable, at times exhilarating, sometimes baffling and disrupting, and it cannot be ignored. The instructor must not only cope with it effectively herself, but enable her student to also cope with it effectively.

• • • • • • • • • • • •

The Goal

Goal is the end to be attained through whatever the practitioner in a practice discipline may undertake. Goal thus is associated with action, to which it gives meaning, focus and justification. In the context of a prescriptive theory, goal is incorporated into the central purpose, but is also recognized as one of the aspects of the realities. As part of the central purpose that enunciates the mission to be accomplished through practice of the discipline, goal specifies the result toward which the practitioner constantly and consistently directs his efforts. As an aspect of the realities, on the other hand, goal specifies the result that the practitioner desires to achieve through the particular activity he currently plans or initiates. Thus, as an aspect of the realities in clinical teaching, goal represents the educational benefit the instructor desires her students to derive from the activities she plans or initiates in their behalf. Such activities might include classes, clinical experiences, individual conferences and assignments of various kinds. The instructor's educational goals might then be said to be, respectively, students' acquisition of knowledge, development of skills, enlightenment regarding some phase of the course and development of insights. By articulating the goal of her educational activity, the instructor gives focus to her action and implies her reason for taking it.

Articulation of an activity's goal does not, however, suggest the way the instructor may go about trying to attain it. Method of attainment is determined essentially by three factors: 1) the central purpose, which influences intent; 2) the framework, which affects ease of application; and 3) the realities, which set limits to execution. It follows, then, that attainment of goal involves three specific steps, each of which has its own particular goal, specifically: 1) goal-in-intent; 2) goal-in-application; and 3) goal in execution.

Goal-in-intent represents the attitude that the insructor believes the student must manifest in order to benefit from the planned educational activity. Consequently, it is an attitude that the instructor needs to consciously foster or engender as part of her effort to attain the activity's goal.

Goal-in-intent derives mainly from the instructor's central purpose which reflects her values and beliefs. If her purpose, for instance, is to facilitate students' efforts to respond capably to the demands the learning activity may impose, her goal-in-intent will most likely be a receptive attitude on the part of students toward the learning activity she has planned. Should her purpose, on the other hand, be to move her students toward independence in their learning and their practice, her goal-in-intent might be a tolerant attitude in her students toward the planned activity. And, should her purpose be to make her students learn what she thinks they need to learn, her goal-in-intent will most likely be an attitude of tractability on the part of her students toward the learning activity she has planned.

The value that students will derive from an activity planned for their learning—a conference, for example, or a class or clinical experience—depends to a large degree on the instructor's clarity about her goal-in-intent and on her appreciation of her need to engender in her students the kind of attitude specified by it *before* engaging them in the activity. If she identifies it, recognizes and respects it, she enables herself to function more meaningfully in her implementation of the activity and she vastly increases the probability of attaining the kind of outcome she desires for her students. On the other hand, if she fails to identify, recognize and respect it, she runs the risk of working at cross-purposes with her students and of having the implementation of the activity defeat the goal she has set for it. For example, during a preclinical experience conference, an instructor whose purpose was to facilitate her graduate students' efforts to respond capably to demands made of them, briefed them on what their responsibilities would be in the clinical area the following day. Her reason for scheduling the clinical experience was to provide opportunity for each student to help a patient according to his experienced need for help. She asked that each student meet her patient, try to establish his need for help and then report back to the instructor before initiating any definitive action. The next day, the instructor noted that one student failed to function as requested, but gave her patient "morning care" without interruption according to her accustomed way. Later, during an individual conference, the student expressed her indignation over having been asked to consult with her instructor about her intended action. That request, she acknowledged, made her feel the instructor had no confidence in her ability as a nurse and she saw no good reason for complying with it. Had the instructor fully appreciated the import of a goal-in-intent, she would have made sure, during the pre-experience conference, that the students understood her reason for the assignment and were receptive to it *before* asking them to carry it out. As it was, at least one student was resistant, with the result that she derived no significant educational benefit from the morning's activity, and the instructor's goal in scheduling the clinical experience was not fully attained.

Goal-in-application represents the kind of framework the instructor believes is essential to the implementation of the educational activity she has planned to initiate. It involves laying the groundwork for the activity so that it may be smoothly carried out by bringing the framework into a supportive relationship with the goal of the planned activity. Goal-in-application is a broad concept that comprehends any and all arrangements and adjustments the instructor must make in order to discharge her teaching responsibilities. Usually, they are more harassing and time-consuming than the actual implementation of the activity. For example, an instructor may wish to hold an individual conference with a student to discuss her progress in the course. She estimates that the conference will involve about an hour of her time; preparation for it, however, might cover days. First of all, she needs to check her schedule to find out what date she could hold the conference. Then she might need to arrange for a quiet place, with privacy assured, in which to meet. This could cause a problem, especially if she shares office space with another instructor whose need to work at her desk might conflict with the instructor's desire to use the office for the conference. Another problem might arise when she tries to make contact with the student—a process which, on occasion, has been known to cover a span of two or three days. Also, when she tries to establish a mutually satisfactory time for the meeting, the student may need to make some personal adjustments and this sometimes cannot be done immediately. Then, when all these facets of the framework have been brought into supportive relationship with her goal in holding the conference, she will still need to take two final steps: 1) obtain from her files appropriate records and other relevant materials she might want to discuss; and 2) notify her secretary that she will be in conference with the particular student at a specified time and place, and ask that she not be disturbed until the conference is ended.

Another example may be found in the arrangements an instructor must make in order to enable her students to have a special type of experience in the clinical area. Knowing that a nurse may possibly be called upon sometime to officiate at a birth, one instructor of maternity nursing wanted to give each of her basic students the opportunity to deliver at least one baby while on assignment in the labor and delivery area. This would be a departure from the labor and delivery experience usually provided students, and, consequently, had to be "sold" to various representatives of the framework, including:

1. The obstetrician-in-chief. This required a special appointment and conference, followed by confirming letter (with carbon copies for the director of nurses and the dean of the school of nursing).
2. The area nursing supervisor. This, too, required a special appointment and conference followed by a confirming letter (with carbon copies for the director of nurses and the dean of the school of nursing).
3. The head nurse on the labor and delivery service. This necessitated a long conference, followed by a letter (with carbon copies for the nursing supervisor and the obste-

trician-in-chief) detailing plans for the students' on-call schedules, for their notification of imminent deliveries by members of the labor and delivery nursing staff and for their responsibilities and relationships to the members of the nursing staff.
4. The senior resident obstetrician and his assistants. This necessitated a conference to advise them of the plans and seek their cooperation and help in implementing them.

Even after all of these arrangements had been completed, the instructor's goal-in-application was still not fully attained. This was brought about only after the students had had their experiences and the instructor had sent letters to members of the obstetric, medical and nursing staffs (with carbon copies to the heads of these services) expressing her appreciation for their help in implementing her plan and the hope that her next group of students might have equally meaningful opportunities and experiences.

Implications of the goal-in-application are far-reaching. It is a significant factor in assuring support from those on whom, to a large degree, successful implementation of a student's learning experience depends. Also, it has potential for laying sound foundations for the future of the program. However, although its recognition is so important to the student's learning, it is often overlooked. It represents behind-the-scenes activities that are apt to be taken for granted; they seldom are made explicit. An instructor's teaching load, for instance, is usually described in terms of actual teaching with no regard for the hours she must spend in making arrangements and adjustments to insure attainment of her goal in teaching. Were goal-in-application accorded full recognition, however, the instructor's "load" would be described in terms of hours spent in teaching *and* in preparation, a practice that would more truly reflect the reality of her commitment.

Goal-in-execution derives from the realities. It represents the degree of supportiveness to the student's potential for learning that the instructor desires the realities to maintain for the duration of a learning activity in order to insure attainment of the activity's goal. The realities consist of the instructor, the students and the framework of the particular learning situation. They are a challenge to the instructor, for they can seriously limit the students' abilities to learn. For example, an instructor who is viewed by a student as a symbol of authority may seem so overwhelming that her presence freezes the student's ability to learn; or, a student may just have fallen in love and her mind is so filled with other thoughts that it cannot take in what is going on; or, the temperature of the room may be so high that the student cannot concentrate on the work at hand. Because of the realities and their limit-setting proclivity, the goal-in-execution may be the most difficult of the three attainment goals for the instructor to reach. To do so calls for vigilance, sensitivity and wisdom all the while that she is engaging in the educational activity: vigilance for signs of negative attitude in any of her students toward the activity; sensitivity to untoward changes in herself or in the framework that could prevent attainment of the activity's goal; and wisdom in dealing objectively and kindly with what she is aware of in the situation so that the student's ability to learn may be supported, restored or enhanced.

The student's behavior during a learning activity will alert the instructor to the degree of interest the activity holds for her. If, when in class, she doodles, dozes or stares into space, her thoughts are probably elsewhere. If she fails to turn assignments in promptly, seems careless in her care of patients or responds truculently when asked to help meet some special nursing need, her behavior strongly suggests lack of receptivity to the activity planned for her learning. Conversely, if the student is attentive in class, makes relevant contributions to discussion, and seeks clarification of a concept that she does not quite understand, then she would appear to be intent on learning. And, if she turns in her assignments promptly or requests a time extension for a reasonable reason, gives seemingly responsible care to her patients and responds willingly when asked to help out in some special way, then her behavior suggests that she is receptive to what she is doing and the instructor may be justified in assuming that the activity is of educational value to the student.

When the student indicates, by her behavior, that she is receptive to a learning experience, the instructor may be said to be reaching her goal-in-execution. When the student gives evidence of lack of interest, that goal presumably is not being reached. Consequently, when a student seemingly is not "with it," the instructor may do well to examine aspects of the realities to see if she can determine the cause of this lack of receptivity. Since the instructor is one aspect of the realities, she might need, first of all, to examine herself, her thoughts and feelings and how they might have been reflected in her tone of voice, manner, words or actions. Quite possibly, her behavior could have given offense. The difficulty could also lie with the student: feelings that may have been hurt; apprehension lest she make an error; worry over something she said or did; headache; weariness; a feeling of nausea. Any one of these conditions could easily be distracting and impair her ability to learn. Other factors of the framework that could be responsible for a student's loss of interest could be: a shortage of supplies the student needs to give the kind of care she might want to give her patient; a poorly ventilated classroom; or the fact that a resident spoke sarcastically to her. Any one of a thousand factors could have a disconcerting effect. Regardless of what the cause may be, it needs to be identified before it can be dealt with. Too, the instructor probably will not feel satisfied with either herself or the course of the activity until she has identified the cause. Once she has uncovered it, circumstances will dictate whether and how to deal with it. Her goal-in-execution, however, is the student's realization of her potential for learning through the activity she is experiencing. This, therefore, must be the true basis for the instructor's decision about what to do to reach that goal.

Goal-in-intent, goal-in-application and goal-in-execution are concepts that are important to effective clinical teaching. Their significance may not always be recognized nor their importance fully appreciated. But when the instructor respects them and makes a determined effort to attain them in her teaching, she is taking a major step toward the realization of her objectives in clinical teaching and the attainment of her educational goal.

● ● ● ● ● ● ● ● ● ● ● ●

The Means

In the context of a prescriptive theory, means are the expedients through which the instructor facilitates students' learning. They constitute the sum and substance of her teaching program. They are the educational activities that both she and her students engage in, and the various devices with which she supplements her teaching and assesses its value to her students. Means include classes, clinical experience sessions, assignments, demonstrations, examinations, and miscellaneous activities such as field trips as well as a wide variety of visual and other aids.

Means serve both the instructor and the students. The instructor may use them as media through which to arouse her students' enthusiasm for the area of nursing they are studying; to give them information that she thinks they may need; and to obtain from them indications of what they know, have learned and are able to do. Students may regard means as opportunities for broadening their horizons and for gaining knowledge, skills and insights essential to the professional practice of nursing. In addition, they may use them as channels through which either to gain clarification and understanding, or to disclose their thoughts and feelings, their knowledge and their skills.

The value that means may have for student learning depends to a large degree on the method of their implementation. This, essentially, is in the instructor's hands. It is her way of conducting classes, not just the fact of class attendance, that arouses a student's interest and enables her to learn. It is the instructor's way of teaching in the clinical area, not just the fact of scheduled clinical experience, that stimulates a student to develop insights that enhance her judgment and her skills in the care of patients. The manner by which means are implemented in an educational program is an individual matter and, to a degree, is unique to each instructor. The substantive topics constituting the content of a program may vary only slightly when outlined by different instructors, but the way they are presented may have wide variations. This is understandable when clinical teaching is recognized as a practice discipline that is guided by a prescriptive theory consisting of a central purpose that gives it direction, a prescription that specifies its fulfilling action, and realities that give it substance, excitement and individuality.

Means encompass a wide variety of activities and devices that will be described in the following paragraphs according to their content and potential rather than their method of implementation. Implementation of the means is recognized as the province of the individual instructor who will activate them as she sees fit. To bring means into focus, however, and make them available for implementation by the instructor, they are presented under five major headings: 1) Classes and Conferences; 2) Clinical Experience in Nursing; 3) Assignments; 4) Tests and Evaluations; and 5) Teaching and Learning Aids. These headings are not mutually exclusive. For instance, conferences are discussed under that heading and also under Clinical Experience in Nursing, of which they are an integral part. But listing the means gives them a degree of organization and so may simplify their use.

Classes and conferences

In the context of clinical teaching, a class may be defined as an assembly of students who have come together for the express purpose of learning about some special subject in which they may be interested or about which the instructor thinks they should know. Class content, for example, could be any subject such as Theory as a Guide to Practice, Nursing Skills, or Anatomy and Physiology. Usually, classes are instructor-planned and dominated, scheduled and somewhat formal. They may be attended by a large or small number of students and their content is apt to be structured and substantial.

A conference, in contrast to a class, is a small gathering of students with an instructor who may, but does not necessarily, dominate it. It may be comprised of the instructor and just one student or it may involve the instructor and several students. Usually, conferences are specially scheduled at mutually agreeable times for the purpose of thinking together and discussing areas of common concern. Thus they tend to be relatively unstructured and informal.

Not infrequently, classes are followed by conferences for those in the group who might like to discuss further some aspect of the class content or who wish clarification regarding its relevance to their clinical area of interest. Thus, conferences, may complement classes and contribute meaningfully to the students' learning.

Among the many ways that classes are conducted is the well-known lecture method, whereby one person gives an informative talk to the students. The speaker prepares his talk in advance and may use anecdotes, freehand drawings on the blackboard, slides, still or moving pictures to illustrate certain points. Most lectures last at least an hour and generally are followed by a question and answer period. All too often, however, that period turns out to be one of verbal exchange between instructor and lecturer, because the students have not yet had time to assimilate what was said and to find out whether they need more information or clarification. While a lecture is in progress, students are usually so busy taking notes that they have relatively little opportunity to do more than hear. If they hear what is said, however, the value of it may come to them after they have had time to review their notes, recall and think about what was said and draw some meaningful conclusions from it. Whether students are receptive to the lecture is seldom apparent and usually no effort is made to find out. Lectures provide opportunities for them to gain special information; the responsibility to *learn* from them is left entirely to the individual students.

Presentations by instructors or instructor-led discussions represent another way of conducting a class. Although they allow for student participation, the instructor leads, and often dominates, the discussion. The content of such classes is relevant to nursing; it consists of information or concepts from which the student may gain insights that will lead to understanding and provide a basis for making valid judgments when giving patient care. Consequently, in addition to leading the class, the clinical instructor has responsibility for obtaining and sustaining the students' interest and involvement.

Advance preparation by the instructor is essential, either for presenting a subject or leading a discussion about it. This involves thorough orientation to the theoretic and substantive components of the subject to be considered, and organization of the material into discussion-stimulating form. The instructor may be able to effect this kind of organization by clarifying for herself her goal in holding the session and by finding answers to questions with the intent of sharing them with her students, for example:

1. Of what interest is the subject to me? or, How did my interest in it become aroused?
2. What makes me think my students might be interested in the subject? or, Of what interest might it be to them?
3. What is my understanding of the subject? or, What is my concept of what all it entails?
4. What do the students think might be the subject's implications for nursing? or, How do they think they might be able to make use of this information in their practice?

By sharing her answers to the first three questions with her students, the instructor may be able to stimulate their thinking and enable them to enter into a thoughtful discussion of the fourth. She may add interest to her presentation if she includes in it accounts of personal experiences and punctuates it with blackboard diagrams or with various visual aids. Students tend to respond positively to examples of real life situations, especially if they can identify with them. A discussion in which students participate in lively fashion is stimulating to both instructor and students. Both she and they may gain from it new ideas and insights that can be put to practical use. Conversely, if the students fail to participate voluntarily in discussion, neither they nor the instructor may derive much value from the class. When the instructor is aware of students' lack of responsiveness, she may do well to try to find out, then and there, the cause of the student's indifference. By sharing her perceptions and assumptions with them—for example, "You seem so quiet today. I'm wondering, is something wrong?"—she may be able to stimulate them to express their thoughts and thus pave the way for holding a worthwhile discussion. Students generally respond enthusiastically to classes in which they can actively participate. They seem to like to have their thinking challenged and to be able to make valid contributions. Many recognize, too, that they need to prepare themselves for the discussions. They appreciate knowing in advance what subject will be considered in class and what relevant preparatory reading they might do.

The seminar is a somewhat sophisticated form of teaching that may be carried on for a selected group of students who are interested in intensive study of some particular clinical problem and related concepts. Students frequently assume the responsibility for conducting a seminar, with the instructor functioning mainly as resource person or consultant. Their study of problems may involve careful search of the literature, community surveys or even setting up pilot programs of some sort in a health agency, in the university or with groups in the community, and usually results in the preparation of a final paper or report.

Clinical experience

As a means to student learning, clinical experience is of greatest value when it is tutorially conducted, and when the student feels prepared to cope with the demands that the realities in the clinical area may place upon her. Clinical experience, thus, needs to be considered in a broad context that includes both the means by which the student may prepare herself for the experience and the means by which the instructor may facilitate the student's learning from it.

REALITIES

The instructor's goal in scheduling clinical experience may be said to be the student's competence in nursing practice. Implicit in this goal is the instructor's desire that the student develop ability to apply nursing concepts and skills appropriately, adequately and economically in her care of patients within the realities of the clinical situation. This suggests that development of competence is a two-pronged process in that it: 1) involves a theoretic orientation to the application of skills that is directed toward grasp of relevant concepts, principles and methods; and 2) includes tutorial experience in practice carried on in a clinical setting. Thus, clinical experience connotes both theoretic orientation and tutorial practice.

Students generally are introduced to nursing concepts, principles and methods through courses consisting of classes dealing with the subject known as Foundations, Fundamentals of Nursing or Nursing Skills. The content of such classes is necessarily broad in scope and general in character. It serves as a basis for practice and may even be an introduction to it; but for application in a particular clinical area, it needs to be refocused and made specific to the realities in that clinical situation. This usually can best be done through pre- and post-experience conferences.

Pre-experience conferences are of two types: 1) those designed to enable students to prepare themselves for practice; and 2) those designed to brief them on their particular responsibilities when in the clinical area.

- **Preparatory conferences**

Preparatory conferences may be one or two hours in length. Their number and content vary according to the students' needs and may include such informative activities as:

- • **A tour of the area**

A tour through the clinical area provides opportunity for students to see it in its entirety and to gain an idea of the location of such important sections as the nursing station, general patient areas, isolation units and the utility, treatment, shower and bath rooms. The tour is more meaningful when it is unrushed and when students feel free to ask questions and to explore such areas as the utility and treatment rooms.

• • Introduction to personnel, policies and practices

Students generally find it helpful to meet, in advance of their actual experience, some of the nurses, doctors and other professionals in the clinical area. Sometimes such introductions can be incorporated in the tour. That is a somewhat opportunistic practice, however, since whom the students will meet depends on who happens to be in the clinical area at the time and is free to be introduced to them. A more reliable arrangement is to ask such various members of the staff as the head nurse, senior resident, social worker and dietitian to meet with the students for whatever length of time may seem appropriate, so that each can discuss aspects of his (or her) responsibilities and the kind of help he (or she) is prepared to give the students. In anticipation of such a meeting and in advance of it, the instructor may want to suggest appropriate areas to discuss. For example, she might ask the head nurse what and where charting is done; how the various record forms are used; how referrals are made to such agencies as the visiting nurse association, the welfare agency or the department of health; under what circumstances it would be appropriate for a student to consult a physician, social worker or dietitian regarding special aspects of a patient's care or rehabilitation. The resident physician might be asked to discuss the conditions, signs and symptoms to be watched for in patients; or the special exercises, treatments or medications that are apt to be prescribed.

• • Rounds

Rounds are a means for acquainting members of a group of the condition of every patient in a clinical area. They may be conducted by actually making the rounds of all the patients, stopping at each bedside to discuss aspects of that patient's condition and care. They may also be conducted as a meeting in a conference room, using the patients' charts as the basis for discussion. Medical rounds are led by the senior resident or by an attending physician for the benefit of the resident staff, interns and medical students. Nurses and nursing students are usually welcome to attend and to participate in them. Their presence gives the doctor opportunity to observe how an individual nurse or nursing student responds to them as well as to the patients—observations that may influence relationships at later times. Such rounds have value for the nursing student, too. They bring her up-to-date on the physical condition of the patients and the medical plans for their care. They also give her a chance to observe the attitudes of different doctors toward patients and nurses, and to become aware of the special interests and concerns they may evince.

Rounds may also be made jointly by the nurse taking charge of an 8-hour period of service and the nurse who has been in charge for the 8-hour period just ending. Such rounds entail an actual visit to each patient and provide opportunity for the charge nurse coming on duty to see all the patients, greet new ones, assess the condition of each and respond to requests, complaints or comments any of them may wish to make. Most charge nurses are quite willing to have students who are new to the area join her in these rounds which can provide meaningful experiences for them. Not only do they acquaint them with all patients in the area, but they also enable them to observe nurse-patient interactions and relations and to gain some understanding of the multiplicity of problems that must be handled by the charge nurse.

• • **Demonstrations**

Demonstrations provide the student with opportunities to observe how a piece of equipment like an autoclave, a resuscitator or an iron lung is manipulated or how certain nursing procedures are carried out. They are accompanied by discussion of the circumstances under which use of the equipment or procedure is appropriate, what the effect of its use might be and what hazards it may entail.

Although the instructor may carry out the demonstration herself, she often asks someone on the hospital staff to do this. For example, if her students are on an orthopedic service, she might ask the head nurse to show them how to bathe or turn a patient who is in traction; and, should they be about to have experience on a medical unit, she might ask the resident physician to demonstrate use of one or more of the cardiac therapy machines.

A demonstration enables a student to visualize as well as understand the functioning of equipment or the implementation of a procedure. This is important to her learning. To develop a degree of confidence, though, in her ability to operate a special machine safely or to carry out a procedure effectively when in the clinical area, she needs to give at least one return demonstration and then to practice until she feels reasonably adept.

• • **Rehearsal for practice within the realities**

Rehearsal for practice is an expedient whereby the student has opportunity to gain insight into her way of interacting with a patient and possibly also into the patient's way of reacting to what the student, as the nurse, may say or do. It is a form of trial practice for a nurse-patient experience within the realities of a clinical situation.

The primary participants in the rehearsal are the students, although on occasion, the instructor may also take part. When she takes the role of nurse, the student is expected to carry out her responsibilities toward her patient in accordance with her purpose in nursing; when in the role of patient, she is expected to appear and act as she thinks a patient with a specified condition might appear and act under the circumstances that have been outlined.

The setting simulates as nearly as possible, a patient unit in the hospital and includes, at least, a bed, a bedside table and a chair. These might be located in an unoccupied area of a clinical unit or in a nursing arts classroom in the school. There needs to be sufficient space for a group of students and the instructor to sit and observe the interaction. A realistic touch is added when the student taking the role of nurse is dressed in nurse's uniform, although a doctor's gown can serve as substitute for the uniform, and when the one representing the patient slips a patient's gown over her uniform or dress.

Orientation of the students to their participation in a rehearsal may take up an entire conference period. This will be time well spent if it results in their understanding not only of the instructor's goal, but also of how the rehearsal may benefit them. A student may feel some reluctance about disclosing her way of functioning to fellow students and instructor, but she may be able to overcome this if she can be helped to view the rehearsal as a means for trying out various approaches and responses and finding out which will be most likely to enable her to obtain desired results.

The situation the nurse is to deal with in the rehearsal is planned in advance and is representative of the kind she can expect to encounter in the clinical area. If her next clinical assignment will be to a medical or surgical unit, the situation would involve a medical or surgical patient; if to a psychiatric unit, it would involve an emotionally disturbed patient; and so on. Facts presented in the pre-rehearsal description of the situation would include the kind a nurse might expect to find on the patient's chart, in addition to other items, as shown in the following example:

Setting: Surgical unit.
Time: 10:00 A.M., February 10, 1968.
Patient: Janet Smith; 29 years old; married.
Appendix removed, February 6, 1968.
Postoperative progress uneventful.
Wants to sign herself out of the hospital because husband has to leave for the Army tomorrow, and her children, ages 5 and 7, need her at home.
Nurse's assignment: General nursing care.

The situation is preferably presented in writing rather than verbally so that a slip describing it may be given to each member of the class, either before or after selection of the students who will take the parts of nurse and patient. Some students appreciate knowing about the situation a day in advance so that they can think out how they might handle the role of nurse or patient. Such preparation has merit, provided the students do not collaborate on a plan of action. In one instance, for example, when two students who were to take the parts of nurse and patient were advised about the situation ahead of time, they planned together how they would develop it. The result was that they put on a performance in which each spoke lines according to the plan they had worked out. It so happened that what they did and said was not fully in relation to the realities of the existing situation. Consequently, they defeated the goal of the rehearsal and felt chagrined when they realized how they had done so.

Situations may be set up by the students or by the instructor. They can allow for more than just the two characters of nurse and patient. They could include, for instance, a head nurse, nursery nurse, nursing supervisor, doctor, instructor or a member of the patient's family. The more characters who are introduced, however, the more complex the situation becomes, and the more difficult it may be to follow the interactions.

Usually, students volunteer for the parts, but if none does, they may be asked to draw lots or the instructor assigns the parts. Each student in the group is expected to enact the role of nurse at least once and, if possible, that of patient at least once, too.

Specific ground rules and instructions for the conduct of the rehearsal should be set up in advance and might include, for example:

1. Decide on the situation that is to be presented.
2. Draw lots for parts.
3. All characters except the patient leave the room, so that:
    a. The room may be readied.
    b. A tape recorder, if one is to be used, may be hooked up and placed.
    c. The patient may place herself wherever she thinks she would be apt to be—in bed, in a chair or away from the area.

4. The instructor and all students not involved in the actual rehearsal seat themselves so that they can all see and hear what the participants do and say during the rehearsal, have pencil and paper handy for note-taking and try to be as unobtrusive as possible during the rehearsal.
5. Nurse (and any other character) advised of readiness to begin.
6. Rehearsal to be carried on for as long as student taking part of the nurse wishes to continue it; the decision to end it rests with her.
7. Critique to follow rehearsal:
   a. Observe a 10-minute period of silence (making notes if desired) for reflection on such questions as:
      1) Did the nurse's approach seem appropriate to the situation with which she was confronted?
      2) Did the nurse try to find out the meaning to the patient of the behavior he presented to her?
      3) Did the nurse identify the patient's need for help before taking definitive action?
      4) Did the nurse meet the patient's experienced need for help?
      5) Did the nurse carry out her assignment?
      6) Was the nurse's action consonant with "good" nursing?
   b. Student who represented the nurse is given first opportunity to comment upon her action and reactions.
   c. Student who represented the patient is given the next opportunity to comment; any other characters then give their comments.
   d. All students and instructor then enter into general discussion.

The discussion during the critique can lead to such valuable outcomes as clarification of concepts, seeing nursing practices in new perspective, or gaining meaningful insights. Effort is made to try to keep it as objective and constructive in tone as possible. Provocative questions that may be raised could be:
how valid are time-honored rituals such as always first introducing oneself when approaching a patient, or always reading a

patient's chart before seeing him? How does the nurse elicit meaningful responses from the patient? How does she motivate a patient to do what may have been recommended when he does not seem to want to do it? During the discussion, suggestions may be made, too, about such things as community facilities to which the nurse may have recourse in her effort to help a patient, or about the many ways by which the nurse can convey to the patient her concern for him and her desire to be helpful.

It may be desirable for students to have·two or three rehearsals before starting their clinical experience in a particular area. This applies not only to undergraduates, but to graduate students as well. Sometimes, the instructor may find it useful to also schedule one or two rehearsals after students have had several experiences in the area. This can be particularly helpful when the situation involves a patient for whom one of the students may have cared, but felt that she did not obtain the kind of results she desired. The opportunity to reenact, for critical review, her way of approaching and responding to the patient can be revealing and valuable.

- Briefing conferences

A briefing conference is a get-together of instructor and students just before the start of a clinical experience session. Decisions are made about which student will care for which patient or patients, previously made plans are confirmed or clarified, new information is presented and pertinent questions answered. Briefing sessions may last as long as half an hour. They have value, even though the students may be functioning as a part of a nursing team and may have already been assigned their patients when attending the nursing staff's morning, evening or night "report" conclave. But by meeting with her students, though perhaps only for a very few minutes, the instructor reaffirms her relationship with them and may be able to deal with, or prevent, problems students and/or she may have or may foresee.

Prior to a briefing conference, the instructor may have made the rounds of the clinical area to assess the general situation. She may also have been able to confer with the nurse in charge regarding how the students might participate in the area's activities. In addition, she may have consulted patients' charts for whatever information they might contain about the patients for whom the students will be caring. The instructor makes advance arrangements with the nurse in charge about the time and place to hold the conference and may also invite her to participate.

- Tutorial practice

Students are provided with clinical experience for a reason. It may be to enable them to develop special nursing skills, to learn how to function in a nursing team, or to gain, through practice, useful ideas on how to identify patients' needs for help or how to cope with the framework of the situation in meeting these needs. Consequently, to insure that what they do in the clinical area will be directed toward the attainment of desired results, the instructor needs to be there, available to them (especially when they are new in the area) and in touch with what they are doing. Her role is essentially that of counsellor, mediator and consultant, but it may also carry some supervisory responsibilities. She is held responsible, to a large degree, for her students' actions and also for the results they get from what they do. Hence, she may need to observe them as they care for patients, see or talk with patients for whom they have cared and read what they have written on patients' charts. Only through firsthand observation can she really learn how her students carry out their nursing functions, and how she can, hopefully, safeguard them and their patients against slips or blunders that could have disastrous effects. She needs such information, too, in order to evaluate her students' nursing practices and to intercede for them, with confidence, should they be criticized or accused.

Students tend to be sensitive and it often takes time for them to tolerate with equanimity the instructor's presence, or to voluntarily avail themselves of the help she is equipped to give.

Time alone, though, does not assure that they will be able to do this. *How* the students experience the instructor is the telling factor and one that depends on what happens in their actual association with her.

Because, in the beginning, students tend to be hesitant about seeking out the instructor for counsel, consultation or help, she may need to take the initiative in making contact with them. Some of the ways she can do this are:

• • By asking each student to confer with her at specific times during the clinical experience period

One such time is after the student has met her patient, has established a relationship with him and has appraised his general condition and state of mind. A conference at this time provides opportunity for the student to give a lucid, focused report about her patient that might include a brief description of him as a person and a concise account of his behavior; her findings on examination or appraisal and her impression of their meaning; and action she may have taken or plan to take. It also gives the instructor an opportunity to appraise the student's understanding of her patient's situation, to discover whether she needs any help and, if so, to offer such help.

Another time for conferring may be before the student does her charting on the patient's record. The entry needs to be informative yet short and to the point. The student may find it helpful to organize her comments under such headings as:

1. Presenting appearance, behavior and/or complaints.
2. Findings upon examination or appraisal.
3. Impression regarding condition or state.
4. Significant action taken.
5. Suggestions for nursing action that may still be needed.

Often students like to make rough drafts of their intended entries, discuss them with the instructor and make whatever adjustments seem appropriate, before recording them on the charts.

Still other times for conferring are before the student tries to carry out a procedure with which she may have had no previous experience, or when she may be baffled by the patient's presenting behavior or by some problem with which she feels she must cope. The instructor's assurance to the student that she is in the area to help and that she is available for consultation may enable the student to seek her out for counsel, should she have such need. If she fails to do so, however, and the instructor becomes aware of the student's need for help, she may need to try to ascertain the cause of her reticence and reluctance to consult and then try to remove it, if possible. The instructor's indifference to the student's ignoring of her presence could lead to further withdrawal by the student and thus defeat the goal of the clinical experience.

- - **By going to the area where the student is giving patient care**

Direct observation of a student's functioning in her care of patients is a means by which an instructor can assess a student's competence and gauge her need for help. Consequently, it is important for her to spend some time with the student while she (the student) is in the process of giving patient care.

Since the instructor's presence in the area may be upsetting to the student, it would be well for the instructor to discuss with her—in advance—her desire to join the student while she is giving care to the patient and thus give the student a chance to suggest how best they might plan for this. Hopefully, the student will also indicate that she is receptive to the idea. In fairness to both the student and the patient, and as a courtesy, the instructor will undoubtedly announce her presence before actually entering the area where the student and patient are. In that way, she can give the student opportunity to invite her to come in. If, however, the student fails to extend an invitation at such time, the instructor may enter the area uninvited and then determine whether it seems appropriate for her to remain. The student may be deeply involved in a conversation that the instructor might not want to interrupt. Or, the student may be in the midst of giving a treatment or carrying out a procedure from which she may feel that she cannot, at the moment, be diverted. Should the instructor sense the student's concentration, she might want to withdraw for the time being, or remain quietly in the area, until the student is free to look up and/or speak. Sometimes her arrival under such circumstances actually is timely, as it was in the incident (see p.   ) in which an instructor entered a patient's room and found the student struggling to insert a catheter. The instructor, though disturbed over the student's fumbling, tried to smile reassuringly at the patient and then went quickly to the bedside. Quietly, she asked the student if she would like her to bring her another catheter and also a lamp so that she could more readily see the meatus. The student, with a wan grin, gratefully accepted the offer. When the instructor returned and focused the light on the patient's perineum, the student was able to see the opening without difficulty. She then inserted the fresh catheter deftly and completed the procedure to the patient's obvious relief.

When engaged in giving some form of patient care, a student may—quite understandably—feel threatened by the instructor's presence. It is important, however, that she try to overcome that feeling because such self-consciousness can defeat her goal in learning as well as in nursing. How to help her sometimes presents a problem. The instructor may find that a prescriptive theory, when understood and applied, will prove its worth in just such a situation. In its context, the student may be able to view the instructor in different perspective, and may be challenged rather than threatened by her presence. She would then regard the instructor as part of the framework, herself as the agent, and her goal-in-application as the need to bring the instructor into supportive relationship with her goal in giving care to her patient (the recipient). When the student understands the implications of her role as agent, her fear of the instructor may diminish. The prescriptive theory, thus, give the instructor a substantive means by which to direct the student's thinking into a realistic channel; it enables the student not only to view the instructor with objectivity, but also to move with clarity toward attainment of her goal.

• • By making opportunistic contact with the student

Another way the instructor can make herself available to students is by circulating in the area and making contact with a student in the hall, at the desk, or in any area other than the patient's immediate vicinity. Such chance encounter can be timely, especially if the instructor greets the student who then may feel free to consult her about some problem she is facing, tell her about some pleasant experience she just had, or ask her for direction or for help.

Circulating and at the same time keeping herself available to all her students is a difficult combination to sustain. It is easier, though generally not as satisfactory, to sit at the desk or in an office and maintain her availability to the students there. But when someone sits behind or by a desk, a degree of formality is introduced into any meeting and this may militate against spontaneity in making comments or requests. When the instructor circulates, however, she may be tempted to become involved in some form of nursing, especially when the clinical area is busy and the nurses seem hard pressed. For instance, a patient may see the instructor and call to her for a bedpan or express some other need; or the instructor may see a patient who seems to be uncomfortable or in distress and feel impelled to try to bring him relief; or a member of the nursing staff or a doctor may try to enlist her aid. Not to respond to such requests may violate her concept of nursing, yet should she respond, she could violate her responsibility to her students. Her decision of what to do will depend on her judgment, based, in all probability, on the realities that obtain at the moment and on who she thinks needs her most. She may be able to respond affirmatively to another's need if doing so will take only a few minutes of her time. Under other circumstances, she might acquiesce, but explain that she needs first to notify her students where she is and how long she will be tied up. Or, she might respond, but with the proviso that should one of her students need her, she would have to interrupt the help she might be giving in order to meet that student's need. Conversely, should she decide not to respond affirmatively, how she says "No" is something that needs to be thought about. Usually, a mere "No" or "I can't" is inadequate. The person asking for help is apt to understand her refusal if she has a valid reason and makes it known, or if she can make a reasonable suggestion of how else, or by whom else, the needed help might be given. Under any circumstances, a request for help should be respected and responded to with candor and concern.

The instructor's need to be in the clinical area with her students may become less acute as they become more confident, able, and less in need of help. However, her need to examine with her students their practice in relation to an explicit prescriptive theory, continues. Such examination may help students to view their actions in clearer perspective and to gain insights that can contribute to the improvement of their nursing skill.

- Post-experience conferences

Post-experience conferences serve several purposes, e.g., to discuss with all students a meaningful experience one of them may have had; to explain, for benefit of all, some policy, facility or procedure; or to stimulate students to think about what they experienced and to identify the factors that enabled them to obtain the results they got from what they said or did.

Ideally, such a conference is scheduled for immediately after the students' experience, while events are fresh in their minds and in the instructor's mind, too. Time may be allowed for it at the end of a clinical session or even included as part of the session, and may last as long as half an hour. Often, however, it is difficult for all students to attend simultaneously and promptly. One may be held up by a patient's last minute request, another by a treatment that is taking longer than she anticipated. Still another might be involved in an interaction with a patient that she feels she can not interrupt. The instructor, too, may be delayed by a student's special need, by a telephone call or by some question the head nurse or a physician may have asked. So that the time of other students who do gather according to schedule will not be unduly wasted, students might be advised ahead of time that, after a certain period of waiting, they should feel free to leave.

A more structured post-experience conference may be held at a later time and deal with analyses of segments of the students practice. Such a conference can be particularly meaningful when students have reconstructed selected sections of their experiences and the instructor has had opportunity to go over their reconstructions before they are discussed. Discussion then can focus on details of the interaction; for example, evidenced respect by the student for her own perceptions, thoughts and feelings; use of communication techniques; and application of nursing principles and concepts. (See pp. 125 ff.) An analysis of a student's reconstruction of an experience she had with a patient may be carried on in different ways and it may be done not only at a group conference, but also during an individual one.

Another way to start a post-experience analysis session is to write on the blackboard the facts about patient's presenting behavior that the nurse perceived, and, when necessary, pertinent background information. Each student then may be asked to indicate, either in writing or verbally, the thoughts and feelings that her perceptions evoked and what action she thinks she might take in response to them.

However an analysis session may be conducted, it usually will be stimulating for the student if it is carried on in an objective, non-judgmental way. It is intended to be a learning experience, one that highlights potential ways of dealing with realities and from which the students may gain insights that they can apply in their nursing.

Assignments

Assignments are tasks that students are expected to carry out, sometimes in groups but more often individually, in conjunction with their courses of study. In a clinically oriented program, assignments may be intracurricular or extra-intracurricular, and they are designed to stimulate the student to develop competence in such functions as thinking, reasoning, creating and applying.

Intracurricular assignments are responsibilities the students are asked to carry out *within* the structure of the curriculum. For example, in a class on Group Process, one student may be assigned the task of leader, one that of observer, and a third that of recorder. Likewise, in a clinical setting, one student might be assigned care of one or more patients and another, the administration of medications. Should the setting be the operating room, a student might be assigned to function as scrub nurse. Preparation for such intracurricular assignments is usually provided within the structure of the curriculum, through such means as discussions, demonstrations or conferences. As a rule, such preparation is general in character and not specific to the particular task. However, when executing an assignment in either area, the student is expected to recall what she learned earlier through discussions, demonstrations or conferences and to exhibit a degree of competence in applying it to the task assigned.

Extra-intracurricular assignments, in contrast, involve responsibilities the student is expected to carry out—usually on her own, but also sometimes in a group with other students—*without* the structure of the curriculum. She is expected, however, to give evidence, *within* the curriculum's structure, of having carried them out. For example, a student might be given a reading assignment that she would be expected to carry out at home or in the library, and then give evidence by her responses in class that she had read what she had been assigned.

Other extra-intracurricular assignments might be to prepare a book review or special report or paper, or to take part in a project of some sort. Each instructor will have her own ideas and will use her own judgment about making assignments that she thinks will have the greatest meaning for her students' learning. She will be guided by such considerations as the amount of time the student might require to carry out the assignment; the reality factors with which the student might need to cope in carrying them out, such as availability or accessibility of facilities; and the student's concomitant involvement in other instructor's assignments. Three types of extra-intracurricular assignments that have been used to good advantage, particularly in Masters programs and which may be of interest to instructors in other types of programs are: a) reconstructions of nursing incidents; b) special projects; and c) summaries of thinking. These three have been selected for elaboration because they are believed to be less widely used than many other types of assignments.

- Reconstruction of nursing incidents

After each clinical practice session, the following assignment might be made: "Prepare a written reconstruction (using special form) of a nursing incident that occurred in the course of your experience in the clinical area and turn it in to me by tomorrow morning. M. Dale."

A reconstruction has been described as follows:

... a reconstruction may be thought of as a rebuilding from memory of an experience the nurse had with a patient, or with someone associated with his care. It is usually in written form, and represents a sequential, detailed description of the nurse's recollection of the patient's (or the individual's) behavior as she perceived it, of the thoughts and feelings which she experienced at the time, and of her ensuing action. It is an attempt to recapture the experience, or portions of it, and to set it down in recalled-image form, so that the elements in it may be identified, examined and appraised in light of her purpose in nursing.

Reconstructions are useful tools-for-learning. To reconstruct necessitates not only recalling details within an experience, but also reflecting upon them, away from the immediate situation in which events often move swiftly, are absorbing, and may allow neither time nor energy for objective examination. Such recollection and reflection often result in insights into one's own motives and action. These insights may add new dimensions to the nurse's knowledge, skills and values that she can apply in the service that she subsequently renders.

To reconstruct an experience takes time and thought. The effort to recall details of the patient's behavior and of the accompanying thoughts and feelings may be considerable, especially if hours have elapsed before making note of them. Details of an experience are most readily remembered immediately after they occur, before the distinctness of their impression has been dimmed by crowding in of succeeding observations, thoughts and events. A tape recording of a nurse-patient experience, when it is possible and feasible to make one, has merit. The recording serves as an aid to memory, because the tape reproduces verbal interaction and the sequence in which it took place. It does not, however, make note of non-verbal behavior which often is more eloquent than the spoken word.

The key to usefulness of reconstruction lies in the detail with which the nurse records the inconsistencies she noted in the behavior of the one with whom she is interacting. If she can recapture the details, she may be able to recall, with a high degree of accuracy, the thoughts and feelings they evoked, and determine where she placed her focus in the action that she took. They also provide a basis by which the reconstruction may be analyzed, and the action appraised in relation to principles of helping, focus and outcome.*

The reason for asking a student to reconstruct a nursing incident is that it forces her to review her action (verbal and nonverbal) and to identify the factors in it that may have been responsible for the kind of results she got from what she did. A reconstruction is a means for learning and thus needs to be, as nearly as possible, an honest representation of what actually occurred. What matters is not so much the outcome of the interaction, although of course it is of concern, but rather the student's recognition of her perceptions, thoughts and feelings and how they influenced her action. The reconstruction of an incident serves actually as a vehicle for presenting the realities in a situation in such a way that the student may examine her overt actions in relation to them. Consequently, she is encouraged to select any sequential incident that occurred. It

---

* Wiedenbach, E., *Clinical Nursing: A Helping Art*. New York: Springer Publishing Co. Inc., 1964.

may be one in which she gained satisfying results or one in which she did not. Either type of incident has potential for valuable learning. To capitalize on it, however, the student needs to review and think about the experience and answer for herself such questions as:

1. Why did I select this particular incident for reconstruction?
2. How did I use my perceptions, thoughts and feelings to identify my patient's need for help or to give the help he needed?
3. What results was I trying to get through what I said or did?
4. What, specifically, did I do or say to get the kind of results I got?
5. What insights into my way of functioning did I get from writing and reviewing this reconstruction?

The five questions on the reconstruction form give the student a focus for her critique. The answers to them give the instructor a clue as to the meaningfulness the reconstruction of her experience had for the student.

Date:_____   Student's Name:_____

College of Nursing, _____ University

Course   Semester   Year

Reconstruction of a Nursing Incident

1. What caused you to select this particular incident for reconstruction?
2. How did you use your perceptions, thoughts and feelings to identify your patient's need for help and/or to meet it?
3. What results were you trying to get through what you did?
4. What specifically caused you to get the results you got?
5. What insights did you gain from writing and reviewing this reconstruction?

(Please give answers at end of reconstruction.)

What I perceived	What I thought and felt	What I did and/or said

126   CLINICAL TEACHING

The following samples are reconstructions of nursing incidents that actually occurred in a number of different nursing settings. They are presented because they bring into focus some of the factors in student-patient interactions that may promote or militate against students' ability to achieve desired results adequately, appropriately and economically.

Reconstruction of Nursing Incident No. 1

What I perceived	What I thought and felt	What I said and/or did
As I entered room and approached the mother, I noted she was in bed, leaning over, having just placed her infant in crib. Straightening up, she adjusted her breast binder by pulling it downward, under both axillary areas. "I'll be glad when I take a shower!"	This behavior, adjusting binder and her words, had some meaning but I don't know what. Should explore to find out.	"How's that?"
"This binder is always riding up under my arms. I feel so warm with it so bunched up." There were indeed many folds of material under her axillae	Perhaps her need is to have binder adjusted.	"Well, it's simple enough to fix that. Maybe I can help you by refitting that binder?"
"I've been thinking of going back to breast feeding my baby."	Inconsistency! Didn't even answer my question. No help to offer to fix binder; wasn't interested. Must be some need here, though, because of her solemn expression and her freedom to converse. But what is the need? Perhaps it does	

REALITIES

What I perceived	What I thought and felt	What I said and/or did
	involve breast feeding. Should persevere along this line and explore it with her. Didn't know she'd been breast feeding.	"Go *back* to breast feeding?"
"Yes. I tried for two days but then decided not to any more and I asked to have baby put on forula."	Wonder what she experienced when she was nursing the baby.	"How did it go when you were trying to breast feed?"
"I was worried the baby wasn't getting enough milk. They told me my milk wouldn't come in for two or three days, but I got scared and thought it would be better if baby got formula instead."	I reacted! Why doesn't anyone stay with primips when they try to nurse their babies? But that's my problem, not the mother's. She's still talking.	
"Then yesterday, sure enough, I did have milk. It leaked out when I was taking my shower, so the nurse put this binder on me. Then last night I started to think maybe I should try to nurse the baby again. But I don't know if I should or not.	Here's an ambiguity.	"How do you mean that?"
I don't know how it will affect the baby." While talking, was fingering bunch of grapes on tray rather aimlessly.	Better explore what she means.	"How do you think it might affect the baby?"

What I perceived	What I thought and felt	What I said and/or did
"Well, I don't know. It might bother her. She's been on formula two days. Now if she goes back on breast—well, maybe it won't work again and then she'll have to go back on formula. All that switching may not be good for her stomach."	This mother needs support in her desire to breast feed. But have I validated that she really wants to nurse baby?	"Do you want to breast feed?"
She looked directly at me. "Yes. I do."	I feel sure she needs support but I think she perceives her unsuccessful attempt as influencing future attempts. Must explore further to find out how she views self and baby in this situation. Both are related to breast feeding.	"Well, how has the baby been taking the formula?"
"O.K."	Explore further.	"She takes enough? And burps? And doesn't seem uncomfortable afterwards?"
Nodding her head after each question. "Yes, she's very good. Goes right off to sleep after I feed her."		"And how did she do earlier when you had her on the breast?"
"She was O.K. I got nervous, though. Thought she wasn't getting enough."	Maybe she needs to understand that she's a good potential candidate for breast feeding.	"Well, then you've got a good feeder in your baby, and you said you noticed you have milk. Seems to me, the baby has what she needs and you have what you need!"

REALITIES

What I perceived	What I thought and felt	What I said and/or did
"And you don't think it will bother her if I nurse her?"	Oh! Will the baby react to the change? Don't really know. How do I share this in a positive way?	"I really don't know for sure. I do think the baby is young enough for a change not to bother her too much."
	Maybe if she knows someone is available to help she might be less worried.	"If you let me, or another nurse, know when it's time for baby's next feeding, one of us will try to be with you to see how it goes."
"O.K. I'll do that."	I remember the mother's mentioning earlier that her left nipple became sore while baby was at breast.	"Maybe while you're in the shower room, I can take a look at your breasts and nipples?"
"That would be fine."		I moved breakfast tray closer to her. "Shall I heat your coffee?"
"No, I usually have to wait till it cools." Made no attempt to eat. Just sat there, fingering breast binder with one hand.	Why doesn't she eat? Inconsistency here. If her need was to discuss breast feeding, surely it's been met. Was her response to my looking at her nipples the clue?	"Would it help if I looked at your breasts now?"
"Oh, yes! That would be fine!" She immediately pushed tray out of way		

What I perceived	What I thought and felt	What I said and/or did
and began to open her gown.	So this is her need for help at the moment—assessment of breast and nipples.	"Good; and while I'm about it, I can adjust the binder and make it a bit more comfortable for you."

In this reconstruction, the student is trying to identify the mother's need for help before giving any help. Although by the end of the interaction the student had gained rather convincing evidence that she had identified the mother's need for help, she probably could have done so in shorter time had she not changed her focus; first she tried to understand the meaning to the mother of the inconsistencies in the behavior she was presenting, then she shifted to trying to learn from her the kind of experience she had had in breast feeding. It is possible that had the student first explored the meaning to the mother of her changeableness regarding breast feeding, she might have learned early in the interaction that the mother was concerned about the condition of her nipples. The student would undoubtedly have inspected the nipples then and there, rather than after the long and somewhat irrelevant conversation that took place.

Regardless of the protractedness of the interaction, however, the reconstruction of it shows that, as it progressed, the student:

1. Showed awareness of the mother's nonverbal as well as verbal behavior.
2. Made deliberate attempts, on occasion, to understand the meaning to the mother of the behavior she presented.
3. Used open-end questions rather consistently in her effort to elicit meaningful responses from the mother.
4. Indicated awareness of inconsistencies in behavior, even though she did not always try to understand their meaning to the mother.

Reconstruction of Nursing Incident No. 2

What I perceived	What I thought and felt	What I said and/or did
Mrs. Klein's arm above the IV needle appeared swollen.	IV fluid must have infiltrated.	Palpated area gently.
	Better lower bottle and see if there's a blood return.	Reached for bottle; looked at patient.
Patient's eyes wide open.	Looks scared to death!	"You look scared. What is it?"
Same expression. Silence. Her eyes were on the IV bottle and tubing.	Is it the IV? This behavior started when I was checking that.	"Is it the IV?"
Same expression. Nodded her head.	What about the IV? Thought of other patients' reactions to IV's.	"What bothers you about the IV?"
Same expression. "Is it all right?"	Remembered when IV was started 20 minutes ago, after two unsuccessful, painful attempts in a small vein above her wrist. She needs an immediate answer. Then I'll pursue reason for reaction.	"I'm checking to see if it's all right." Continued to check. Adjusted tape on needle; exerted pressure; finally got good blood return; put bottle back on pole. "It seems O.K. now. I wanted to make sure the needle was in your vein so you'd get the fluid."

What I perceived	What I thought and felt	What I said and/or did
Relief flowed over her face. The original expression faded. Smiled.	What did this mean to her? Why was she so scared?	"What was there about the IV that frightened you so?"
Smiled. "I wasn't scared—it's all right."	Inconsistency between her words and facial expression.	"Your facial expression made me think you were scared and it seemed to be something about the IV. I just wondered what it was and wanted to see if there was anything I could do to help."
Smiled, then an expression of fright flashed across her face. She whispered: "I was afraid it wasn't all right and they'd have to try again. It hurts so much when they do that." Closed her eyes. Went to sleep.		

This reconstruction exemplifies the importance of maintaining awareness of the patient's behavior when carrying out a technical procedure in her behalf. Specifically, it shows how the student identified and met her patient's need for help by:

1. Sharing with the patient her perceptions of inconsistencies in the patient's appearance and behavior.
2. Persevering in her effort to understand the meaning to the patient of the behavior the patient presented to her.
3. Indicating in her action, her respect for her own perceptions, thoughts and feelings.
4. Obtaining validation from the patient that her need for help had been met.

REALITIES   133

Reconstructing of Nursing Incident No. 3

What I perceived	What I thought and felt	What I said and/or did
"Would you get me a pill? I have a pain down here." Points to lower abdomen.	Probably afterpains.	"What does it feel like?"
Couldn't explain.	Still thinking in terms of afterpains.	"Is it crampy, sort of? Like menstrual cramps?"
"Yes, ma'am."	I'll check all possibilities.	"May I check first? There might be something else I can do to make you comfortable."
"O.K."		Palpated abdomen.
	Fundus firm. Bladder could stand to be emptied; may need enema.	"Would you like to go to the bathroom? That may relieve your pain."
"All right." Went to bathroom. I saw two bottles for "peri" care sitting on her stand.	She doesn't know about peri care on her fourth day?	Took bottles to her. "You forgot these. Did anyone show you how to use them?"
"No ma'am."	It's important that she know this. She has stitches.	Showed her how to do peri care. "This will keep your stitch area clean and that's important so you won't get an infection."
"Yes ma'am."	Give her a reason she will like better.	"If you use nice warm water, it'll make your stitches feel better." Demonstrated.
"That does help."		"Good. Use this everytime you go to the bathroom, and change your pad each time. These little tissues are to dry off with."

What I perceived	What I thought and felt	What I said and/or did
Back in bed.		Palpated abdomen.
	Fundus firm. Two fingers below umbilicus. That's better.	"Is your pain any better?"
"No ma'am."	Feels as though bowel may be full.	"Was your bowel movement yesterday a good one?"
"No. Just a little."		"Would you like an enema?"
"Yes ma'am."		Gave her an enema, then palpated abdomen.
	Good results. Abdomen feels less gassy.	"Feel better now?"
"It still hurts here." Points to right side of lower abdomen.	Muscles. That's it, of course! I shouldn't have suggested to her it was a crampy pain.	"I'll get your pill in a minute. Would you like to learn some little exercises to help you get your figure back and tighten these muscles that ache.
"Yes ma'am."	She's anxious to learn exercises.	Showed her exercises.
	Cooperates well.	"You can do those every hour and you'll soon find your muscles feeling much stronger. Do you still need a pain pill?"
"Yes, please. It hurts here." Pointed to both sides, lower abdomen.	She doesn't seem really in pain, but is probably uncomfortable.	"I'll be right back with it." Left room.

This reconstruction exemplifies nurse-directed action. Although the student carried out a number of nursing procedures such as palpating the mother's abdomen, feeling for her fundus, giving her an enema, demonstrating postpartum exercises and, finally, getting her a "pain pill," she did so without endeavoring at any time to identify, deliberately, the mother's experienced need for help. Specifically, the interaction reveals that the student:

1. Asked primarily closed end questions (leading to "Yes" and "No" answers).
2. Indicated awareness of verbal behavior almost exclusively.
3. Suggested to the mother how and what she may be feeling; how and what she should do; and presented no evidence that the mother was receptive to her suggestions.
4. Acted in response to her own unvalidated assumptions of the mother's need.
5. Gave no evidence of having obtained validation that the help she assumed she gave, was experienced as help by the mother.

- Special projects

Special projects comprise investigative or developmental activities in which one or more students are asked to engage. They usually involve intensive study and tangible expression of outcome. Special projects are demanding. The student is expected to invest a substantial amount of time, energy and effort in her project and she usually is encouraged to select its subject herself.

Projects that students may undertake are legion in number and variety. They may involve creating something; searching the literature as a basis for presentation of a paper; engaging in some kind of research; developing a community action program; or leading a class discussion on some timely subject. A few examples of special projects follow:

1. A group of students wrote and presented a play portraying a public health nurse's home visit to a family to persuade the mother, in accordance with the doctor's recommendation, to have her youngster's tonsils removed. The family had social as well as other health problems. The audience for the play included fellow students, faculty members, physicians, representatives from the local visiting nurses association and hospital nurses.
2. Another group of students fashioned a model uterus and adnexa from pieces of silk, foam rubber and fine yarn, and fitted it into a model female pelvis. Execution of the project called for search of the literature, examination of anatomical displays, ingenuity and creativity. It also necessitated preparation of a paper describing the process of fashioning the model, its salient features and suggestions for its use.
3. A group of senior students were assigned to carry out, individually, the systematic investigation of some nursing problem, for example, "The effect of an experimental process of nursing on patients' perception of tension;" and to present a report of it to fellow students and members of the faculty.
4. A student developed a series of community and family health education classes for graduate students and their wives in a university community, and presented a report on the organization, development and results of that undertaking.
5. Each of a small group of students was asked to conduct a class discussion on a subject of her choice but related to the clinical specialty in which she was involved. Her classmates participated in the discussion that was to be conducted in the context of a prescriptive theory. This assignment entailed not only careful search and review of the literature and visits to local agencies, but also special organization of material for the discussion, and this proved to be a challenge. It meant that she had to:
   a. Clarify for herself and make explicit, her central purpose in leading a discussion on the particular subject she had chosen.

REALITIES

b. Justify her assumption of the role of discussion leader.
c. Decide upon the way (prescription) that she would try to conduct the discussion.
d. Recognize the realities in the situation and their implications:
   1) The agent—herself. As agent she would need to specify for herself what she thought her commitment might be with respect to leading the discussion.
   2) The recipient—her classmates whom she would lead in discussion. She would need to decide whether she regarded them as potentially capable, essentially capable or incapable of participating in the discussion.
   3) The framework—the actual setting, with the instructor as part of it. As agent she would need to decide, too, whether she regarded the total framework and/or its various parts as potentially supportive, essentially supportive or nonsupportive.
   4) The goal. She would need to specify for herself what she hoped the outcome of the discussion would be:
      a) Her goal-in-intent—the kind of attitude toward the discussion she would try to engender in her classmates (the recipients).
      b) Her goal-in-application—the kind of supportiveness toward attainment of her goal, that she would try to effect in the framework (including the instructor).
      c) Her goal-in-execution—the kind of attitude and/or supportiveness toward her goal she would try to sustain within the realities for the duration of the discussion in order to insure attainment of the goal.
   5) The means—all the expedients she might use in order to have the discussion move along smoothly and effectively. They would include knowledge about the subject to be discussed and the special

skills she would be expected to display in leading the discussion, reading material she might want to suggest, mimeographed material she might want to distribute, seating arrangements she might think appropriate, lighting effects, visual and other aids and, possibly, resource persons she might want to invite to be present.

As a rule, such projects are intended to summarize aspects of a student's learning in a particular course of study. An instructor may be asked to serve as the student's advisor, but usually the actual development of the project, its preparation for presentation and the presentation itself are strictly the student's own.

- **Summaries of thinking**

Summaries of thinking are written, personal exchanges between student and instructor. The instructor asks each student to turn in at stated intervals (sometimes as often as every week), a summary of her thinking about her learning experiences to date. She may suggest, too, that the student emphasize such aspects as the insights she thinks she gained, clarification she might need, and factors that she thinks promoted, supported or impeded her ability to learn. The instructor responds in writing to each student's summary. In this way, she is able to maintain an individualized relationship with each student and has a medium through which she can give special help or encouragement.

Usually, students require a few experiences in writing summaries and in receiving the instructor's replies before they seem able to write them with candor and to use them as a means by which to enhance their learning. At first they tend to give general impressions without indicating the significance to them of their impressions. Students may write, for instance, "The class on concepts was interesting. It gave me some new ideas to think about." Such a comment suggests that the student has been thinking about her experiences, but it does not indicate what special meaning they had for her. Consequently, in her response, the instructor may ask the student, "Just what about the concepts class did you find interesting?"

Gradually, however, the students' summaries become more revealing of their insights, reactions, confusions, questions and aspirations. In them, students lay bare their thoughts and thus give the instructor opportunity to respond directly to these thoughts. For example, one student wrote:

"At present, I am very confused about what I think I should be doing for these patients. I think the class on principles of helping was very good because it helped me see what I should have been trying to do, yet I am very confused when I try to integrate these ideas with the other ideas I have about nursing care. Perhaps the solution would be to throw my old ideas out and start over again, but I cannot do that."

To this the instructor responded:

"You were not alone in feeling confused and frustrated by your first morning on the unit. It did show up gaps between theory and practice, and made you take a close look at theory in relation to practice to see how valid it is. It also made you take a close look at your performance to see if you really did help the patient you were caring for. So, although the experience was not particularly satisfying to you, in retrospect, I think some pretty useful things came out of it for you, in a learning context.

"Indeed, I hope you throw out nothing that you have learned to date. You have a good background. We want to build on it; not displace any part of it. So, hang on to what you have and try to see what you can add to it to make it stronger."

Included in another student's summary was the following paragraph:

When I think of my progress to date it's difficult to believe that we are already at midsemester. My nurse-patient interaction, I feel, is generally pretty poor. There is so much to improve. For one thing, I still don't realize my reactions to a patient's presenting behaviors until much later, after the interaction. So many things come to mind when I'm reconstructing a situation. And then so much more comes to light during conference when we go over the interactions. When will I be able to do at the time of the interaction that which I do in a reconstruction?"

The instructor's response was:

"The midyear period seems a long way off at the beginning of the year, but then—all of a sudden—it is here. Like now! And, when you try to take stock of what you actually have accomplished in this time, you may well feel some disquieting moments—that is, if you expect to have achieved complete clarity of vision and competence in action.

"The learning process isn't that simple or that fast. It involves self-awareness, acquisition of ideas, insights, practice, reflective thought, self-awareness again, new insights, more practice, more reflective thought, over and over again. In fact, when you really are interested in improving your practice, this cycle goes on and on and on!

"You have made a good start on the cycle. You most certainly have gained self-awareness; you have acquired some useful ideas; you have developed insight into your use of self and the effect that what you do often has; and you reflect purposefully and analytically on what you do. That you may need help to analyze more fully is not unusual. Most of us do. We just aren't so self-sufficient that we can figure out everything, completely, unaided, always. Even with help, we don't always do the figuring out job completely."

Another student wrote, among other things:

"I have been trying to look at my own behavior and my reactions to others and to situations. I do see some pattern, I think. And reactions that I suppress do pop out at the most inopportune times. I am most afraid of getting angry at someone, but I do, and it is best that I acknowledge the feelings that I have and try to understand what precipitated them. I was angry with Jane this week, as I have been in previous weeks. She kept asking me what I thought about things and I didn't want to tell her because I didn't think it would be appropriate in relation to what she was feeling and thinking. I listened to her for quite a long time and told her my opinion and that I wondered what she wanted from me. She accused me of being 'deliberative'."

To this, the instructor responded:

"Anger is a form of reaction and you need to try to find its cause and check the validity of its base, if you want to deal with it usefully. If Jane kept asking you things you didn't want to answer, maybe you should have tried to find out how come she kept asking you how you felt about this or that. The anger you felt might have alerted you to the fact that you didn't understand her reason for asking you, and so her asking didn't make sense to you.

"When she accused you of being deliberative, did you take that as an insult or as a compliment?

"If you have a lot of pent-up anger, it would seem to me a good idea to try to talk about it. It's not good to any one, bottled up, and could explode!"

Still another student wrote:

"I have been approached by one of the psychiatric nursing students with the statement that 'Psychiatry is *the* place for capturing and understanding deliberative nursing, if you're going to learn it, because in psychiatry you have more time, without hospital routine and nursing procedures, to talk to and simply be with the patient.' I disagreed because I think deliberative nursing can be effective in all nursing no matter what the area or the type of nursing one does. Also, I do not see carrying out a treatment as a necessary hindrance to understanding the deliberative art: I can still hear, see and talk even if my hands are busy. . . . I'd like your opinion concerning psychiatry as *the* place for deliberative nursing."

The instructor's response to that section of the student's summary was:

"Every student when challenged, will strongly defend the area of her special interest. And even when not challenged, may at some time feel the need to justify her choice. This is fine when it isn't done at the expense of another student's area of interest.

"When a psychiatric nursing student says that psychiatry is the best area in which to learn how to nurse deliberatively, I certainly would want to know how she means this. That's a very ambiguous comment that I could interpret in several ways, three ways to be exact. Is the interest in nursing, in psychiatric nursing, or in being deliberative?

"If it is nursing, then the focus will be on identifying the patient's need for help, on providing help needed, and validating that the help provided met the need for help experienced by the patient.

"If it is psychiatric nursing, then in addition to the focus on the three components of nursing, focus will also be on development of resources for identifying and meeting needs for help experienced by mentally disturbed patients.

"If it is on being deliberative, focus will be on recognition of the ambiguity inherent in another's behavior, and effort will be directed toward gaining clarification of the meaning to the other of his behavior or confirmation of our interpretation of it, before taking any definitive action such as giving information or some other form of help.

"Ambiguities may be more obvious in the behavior of mentally disturbed patients. Those of you who elected to specialize in maternal and newborn health nursing, however, would not be benefited particularly, in the time available, by having clinical experience in a psychiatric area. It seems much more appropriate to have it in the obstetric area, where behavioral ambiguities may seem less exaggerated but nevertheless exist, and where the needs experienced by the patients support the development of your resources for identifying and meeting those needs."

Responding to students' summaries of thinking is provocative and time-consuming. The written dialogue, however, allows for a personal exchange of thoughts between student and instructor, and many times results in revelations that are important to the instructor's understanding as well as to the student's learning, and that otherwise might not have come to light.

Tests and evaluations

Tests and/or examinations are generally assumed to be expedients for determining the extent of a student's knowledge, understanding and/or skill with respect to a special area of interest, or for gauging her potential for safe and competent functioning in such an area. They are time-honored devices, upon which a wide variety of agencies depend, to a large degree, for implementation of their policies on admission, promotion and, in educational institutions, graduation as well. Such agencies include colleges and universities, professional schools, state boards of examiners, civil service agencies and a host of business, industrial and professional organizations.

Tests may be thought of as having two potential uses: 1) as a measure of knowledge and competence; and 2) as a teaching tool.

As a measuring device, the value of tests is subject to question. Inherent in them are serious limitations that would seem to militate against attainment of an important goal of education, namely, preparation of an individual for life situations. Some characteristic limitations of tests or test questions are:

1. They are generally unalterable. They usually cannot be elaborated or interpreted, even when not fully understood by the one being examined.
2. They often seem to encourage "tunnel vision." They generally call for specific answers which at best represent only a fragment of a student's knowledge, understanding, skill or potential for functioning.
3. They tend to be one-dimensional. They are apt to call for "Yes" or "No" answers and make little if any allowance for possible extenuating circumstances or exercise of judgment.
4. Regardless of kind, they are inevitably presented in hypothetical context. Thus, of necessity, they exclude significant aspects of the realities that are so important a part of life situations.
5. They tend to produce anxiety in the individual taking the test. This can obfuscate her vision and impair her ability to think.

As a teaching tool, however, tests may have merit, for they can contribute in several ways to a student's learning:

1. They accustom the student to taking examinations—an experience that could stand her in good stead in the future when her acceptability for employment or advancement may depend upon her ability to pass a test creditably.
2. They motivate the student, in anticipation of taking an examination, to review her notes, relevant textbooks and procedures, and thus help her not only to fix facts and concepts more firmly in her mind, but also to gain new insights and understandings that might have been lost to her had she not undertaken such review.
3. They motivate a student to study and to practice daily—particularly when they are "sprung" at frequent intervals throughout a course—and thus enhance as well as keep current her knowledge, understanding and skill.
4. When conducted as an oral group activity, they cause the student to "sharpen her wits," and heighten her ability to "think on her feet" and to give clear, concise focused responses to oral questions. These abilities may also stand her in good stead in the future when working in interdisciplinary situations.

Tests and examinations may be written or oral, announced or unannounced, practical or theoretic, midterm or final. What kind to include in a clinical teaching program, when and how often to give them and even whether to give one at all, are generally decisions the instructor is expected to make. If she decides to give one, however, she usually is responsible for its construction, unless she makes use of a ready-made test that may be available through such a source as the National League for Nursing.

The decision to construct and give a test presumes that the instructor has considered five questions:

1. What is the goal of the test or examination?
2. What will be its format and content?
3. How will it be administered?
4. How will it be scored?

5. How much weight, with respect to the student's course grade, will be attached to the score?

The goal that the instructor envisions for the test will give direction to the decision she makes about its format and content. Assuming that she regards tests as tools for student learning, the goal would be the value to the student, as well as to herself, that she hopes to effect through use of that tool. For example, it might be a summarization of the salient aspects of the course to date; it might be the revealment of areas in the student's learning that need clarification or reinforcement; or, it might be identification of areas in course content on which the instructor might want to place her emphasis next or in the future. The instructor's reaction to realities in her current teaching situation are often the factors that influence her in her determination of a test's goal. She may be concerned over students' abilities to keep up with the rate of speed with which the course has been moving, or over the volume of material covered in it, to date. She may be dismayed over the quality of students' responses to situations confronting them in class or in the clinical area, or uncertain about the extent of students' grasp of the meaning of concepts and their implications for care of patients. Each test that an instructor gives will, of course, have an outcome of some sort, regardless of whether the instructor has specified its goal. When none is specified, however, the outcome is left to chance and may not allay or justify her concern or answer her questions. On the other hand, when the instructor makes the goal explicit before attempting to design the test, and lets it influence her in its construction, she not only gives focus to the examination, but also assures, to a high degree, that the test will provide information that she may use, directly or indirectly, to further the students' learning, in meaningful, optimum fashion.

Format and content are the real substance of a test or examination. Format represents its nature and general arrangement; content, the actual questions or problems posed. Although the instructor has a wide choice in each, the two are interrelated. The format she decides upon places limits on the content she may use, and the content she decides upon places restrictions on the format she may use. For example, she may have decided to give an oral examination but she also wishes to use multiple choice questions and, since this type of question is inappropriate in an oral examination, she would need to change the format to that of a written one.

Because written examinations must be responded to in writing, they do not lend themselves readily to group activity, while oral ones do. Questions, problems or problem situations for either type of test may be presented to the students in written form, using paper or blackboard, or they may be read to the students by the examiner. They may also be presented by means of some audiovisual device as video tape, films of some sort or playback of a tape recording.

Outlining the test instructions and formulating the questions needs to be a thoughtful undertaking because students are expected to accept them at face value and to respond directly to them. Consequently, their clarity and freedom from ambiguity is a major consideration. Their meaning is usually more easily grasped when they are succinctly stated, couched in simple language, and only one thought is included in each test question or part of a question. For example, the instruction, "Describe and discuss the local application of dry cold" would probably be more easily understood and yield more cogent responses if it were presented in parts and elaborated to read:

  A. Describe the procedure *local application of dry cold* with respect to:
    1. Appropriate materials the nurse might use to carry it out.
    2. Essential steps the nurse must perform to accomplish it.
  B. Discuss the procedure from the following aspects:
    1. Its potential effect on the patient;
      a. Physical
      b. Physiological
      c. Psychological
      d. Chemical

2. Circumstances under which application of dry cold would be indicated.
3. Circumstances under which application of dry cold would be contraindicated.

Compound questions or instructions that are broken up in such fashion are more easily scored than they are when their parts are not separately identified.

Another consideration in constructing examination questions is their relevance to whatever the students may be expected to know, to conclude or to be able to do, on the basis of their experiences in the course to date. Still another consideration is the time that may be required to complete the test. The number of items to which students would be expected to respond should be realistic with respect to the amount of time available for the examination. Thus, the complexity of the questions and of their anticipated answers are factors to keep in mind. A student's response to the "local application of dry cold" instruction just cited, could be expected to take considerably more time than one called for by such a question as: 1. a) What is molding? b) What is the significance of molding to labor?

All such considerations suggest another important facet of test construction, the recording, for use as a standard, of the correct answers to the questions, or at least the essential information which the instructor thinks the responses should include. Then, when she has completed construction of the test, the instructor may find it helpful to try out her test questions and/or instructions, ahead of time, on a colleague who is knowledgeable about the subject, the plan of the course, and the students' progress in it. If her colleague thinks that the questions are clearly stated and relevant, that their meaning may be easily grasped, and that their number is realistic in relation to the allotted time, then the instructor may feel reasonably secure in her assumption that the students will be able to understand the questions and that the test's goal will be attained. If, on the other hand, her colleague thinks that the questions are ambiguous, irrelevant, too simple, too complex, too many or too few, then the instructor may want to make adjustments in the examination before submitting the questions to her students.

Tests may be administered in a number of ways. The method determined upon will depend, in part, on what the instructor desires her students to gain from it as well as what she, herself, hopes to gain. In other words, the method she uses will depend on the goal that she may envision for the test in the context of the realities of the situation.

If she wants to accustom the students to taking examinations and at the same time gauge their assimilation of facts or their understanding of concepts, she might have the questions typed, duplicated and then distributed to the students in class, where they will write out their answers. If she wants them to enhance their familiarity with library resources and appraise their competence in using such resources, she might give the students questions to answer "out of class," but with the understanding that they neither consult each other nor compare their answers or the sources they used in arriving at them. If the instructor desires to motivate the students to develop habits of daily study and, at the same time, to gauge the degree of their understanding of subject matter, she might "spring" quizzes at frequent intervals throughout the term. If she desires to give the students opportunity to "think fast on their feet" and at the same time estimate their grasp of concepts or of facts, or the students' understanding of the relevance of concepts and facts to practice, she might give a "spelling bee" type of examination, or one resembling a "College Bowl"* performance. Because they are oral, these two types of examinations have the advantage of enabling the students to strengthen their knowledge on the basis of each other's answers, regardless of whether those answers are initially correct. A "College Bowl" type of test, in contrast to the spelling bee type which may be given to a relatively large number of students, lends itself best to examination of a small group. A total of six might be considered a maximum number, and three the minimum. Three judges who are knowledgeable about the subject will need to be appointed.

---

* Adapted from the "College Bowl" program which has been presented on television over channels of the National Broadcasting Company.

REALITIES 149

The instructor may want to serve as moderator. Questions are prepared ahead of time and listed on separate cards each of which is numbered, prominently, on its back. If the instructor wants the questions to be comprehensive, she may fit them into such categories as *Definitions, Facts* and *Situations.* The number of questions assigned to each category should exceed by at least one or two the number of students being examined so that each student, including the last one to be examined, will have a choice of questions. Thus, if three students are being examined, the number of questions per category, would be at least four. The question cards may then be grouped according to categories and displayed in such a way that their numbers, not the questions themselves, are visible. The procedure for such an examination might be as follows:

1. Students, seated or standing, are asked to line up.
2. Students are asked questions individually, in clockwise rotation, beginning with the student who either volunteers to be the first, or who is designated by the moderator to be the first.
3. Each student may select her own question, by card number, from the category specified by the moderator.
4. After a student has completed answering the question, her answer is scored by each judge.
5. Each remaining student, in clockwise rotation, is then given opportunity to contribute facts or relevant information not yet presented. Any student making such a contribution is given credit on her score according to the validity of her reply.
6. If a student is unable to answer a direct question, she is considered to have *failed* the question and receives a score of zero. The question is then offered to the next student in line. If she answers the question, her answer is scored by the judges and then the remaining students are asked to contribute any relevant additional points they may have thought of, according to procedure 5.
7. The student next in turn to the one who answered the "failed" question is the next one to select a question.

8. The examination continues until each student has had opportunity to answer a direct question that she selected from each category.

Scoring of tests, regardless of the kind they may be, can be a relatively simple matter or it can be complicated. The simpler the process is kept, however, the greater will be the validity and objectivity of the score. Two factors, especially, contribute to ease in scoring. One is to ask questions that call for simple answers. The other is to make a list of answers that the instructor considers to be the correct ones, before administering the test, and give it to whomever will score the answers.

Questions that call for simple answers include the kinds that may be answered by "Yes" or "No," a numerical figure, one or two words, or a single statement; for example the various kinds of multiple choice questions, mathematical problems, and questions or instructions asking for definitions. Answers to such questions are either correct or incorrect, so that a single score may be given to each. What that score may be depends on the scoring system the instructor has adopted. If she uses a system involving a scale of 0-100, she would divide the number of questions into 100, and the result will equal the score to be assigned to each correct answer. Compound questions can be made relatively simple, too, and each part treated as a "simple" question or instruction and given its individual score. Since whole numbers are easier to work with than fractions, scoring will be simplified if the total number of questions asked can be divided evenly into 100 and if the number of parts of compound questions can be evenly divided into the score value assigned to the total question.

If, in advance of administering a test, the instructor lists the answers that she considers correct for each question, she, or whoever acts as judge, can use them as a standard when assessing the correctness of the students' answers. When questions are simple, their correct answers can generally be readily determined; but when they are compound, determining their correct answers may be more difficult. This is especially true of situational type questions such as: "A baby, weighing 1400 grams, is admitted to the special care nursery and placed in your care. a) What characteristics would it probably display? b) What might be your course of action? c) What would be your reason for taking it?" Rather than specifying firm answers that the instructor might consider correct for each part of the question, she might specify the essential points that she thinks should be included in the answers; for example; a) descriptive statements about the baby's color, cry, breathing, heart beat, muscle tone and appearance of body; b) comments about such actions as evaluating the baby's condition, dealing with the mother's reactions and consulting or reporting to the physician; c) the student's justification for each action listed. If the student includes in her responses not only the points the instructor considers essential but other points as well, each "other" point may be recognized by a bonus score that should, however, be of lesser value than that assigned to each essential point.

How much weight, in relation to the final grade for the course, to attach to examination scores is a question the instructor usually must answer herself; and her decision is apt to be an arbitrary one. Much depends on the importance she attaches to examinations. If she thinks of them as devices for measuring students' knowledge or competence, she probably will attach more weight to them than she would if she regarded them as teaching tools. An instructor, for example, who specifies that students' final course grades will be given on the basis of such activities as midterm and final examinations, seminar presentations, periodic quizzes and satisfactory performance in laboratory assignments, probably regards examinations as measuring devices. So, too, might the instructor who, in determining a student's final grade, assigns a weight of 45 per cent to examinations, 5 per cent to written assignments, and 50 per cent to clinical performance.

On the other hand, an instructor who regards examinations as teaching tools will use them to promote students' learning. She therefore will probably attach the same weight to an examination score that she would to a score given for any other learning activity. She might, however, differentiate, with respect to weight, between a quiz and a final examination. For example, should she use a score form similar to the sample presented here she might regard a student's quiz score as an indicator of an attribute such as Understanding; but regard the final examination as a complete learning situation. In that event, the score of the final examination would replace the sum of scores assigned to the various desirable attributes manifested by a student in other types of learning situations. Thus, the quality of a student's participation in several successive learning situations, including a quiz and a midterm examination, might be scored and evaluated as indicated on the sample score sheet (see next page).

No ideal evaluative system has yet been evolved. The instructor must use her own judgment in determining how she can best arrive at fair grades for her students. If she can incorporate a learning opportunity into the evaluative process, her students are apt to welcome it. If she treats a final examination not as a major index of their competence but rather as just another learning stiuation, her students may undertake it with a degree of confidence, unhampered by the fear or anxiety which all too often impairs the quality of their responses.

Teaching and learning aids

Teaching and learning aids comprise the whole range of items and equipment that are recognized appurtenances of an educational program. Some of them, like pens, pencils and erasers, chalk, paper clips and rubber bands, may have little intrinsic value, but not to have them when they are needed could cause the instructor or the student to feel seriously handicapped. Tables, desks, chairs, blackboards, scrap baskets and other furnishings that are in daily use are all means that serve both a teaching and a learning end, and their availability to both student and instructor is generally taken for granted.

Other types of teaching and learning aids include record players, tape recorders, moving picture and slide projectors and audiovisual machines. Although costly, they are in wide use

REALITIES 153

Course: _____ Student: __Mary Ann Dow__

Semester: __Second__ Year: __1969__

Minolta University
Score sheet for Evaluating Student Participation in Learning Situations

ATTRIBUTE	SCORE	Ed. Activity: Clinical Experience Date: 4/11/69
Constancy in Purpose	C = 1	Concentrated on social Substantiating facts: problems; forgot physical evaluation. Described inconsistencies but not clear about what to do with them. No effort to ascertain patient's receptivity to intended action. Made excellent suggestions for follow-up by VNA. Concerned about state of ward and recognized its inherent realities; sought help in thinking through how to deal with them.
Understanding	C = 1	
Competence	B = 2	
Deliberateness	C = 1	
Responsibleness	B = 2	
Resourcefulness	A = 4	
Score, total: 11 av. 11/6 =1 5/6 = C		Instructor: O. J. Smith

ATTRIBUTE	SCORE	Ed. Activity: Class: Ng. theory Date: 4/14/69
Constancy in Purpose	C = 1	Sprung quiz: B Substantiating facts: Digressed when something reminded her of some unrelated past experience; gave lengthy account of it:(A former student who failed to report a high BP when in the clinical area). Sought clarification re levels of theory. Tended to generalize and stereotype:"All nurses are careless about charting. They don't report findings."
Understanding	B = 2	
Competence	B = 2	
Deliberateness	D = -1	
Responsibleness	C = 1	
Resourcefulness	—	
Score, total: 5 av. 5/5 = 1 = C		Instructor: M. Jones

ATTRIBUTE	SCORE	Ed. Activity: Mid-term exam. Date: 4/15/69
Constancy in Purpose	—	Substantiating facts: Prompt in arrival for exam. Attentive to instructions; seemed to concentrate on questions until finished. Wrote legibly. Situational examination questions.
Understanding	B = 2	
Competence	—	
Deliberateness	—	
Responsibleness	A = 4	
Resourcefulness	—	
Score, total: 6 av. 6/2 = 3 = B		Instructor: F. R. Brown

Directions for scoring:

Score Symbols:
A = 4 Range: 3½ - 4
B = 2 Range: 2 - 3½
C = 1 Range: 1 - 2
D = -1 Range: -1 - 1

Assign quality symbol to each indicator of an attribute and convert symbol into appropriate number value. Add numbers and divide sum by total number of indicators evaluated. Result equals score for participation in that particular learning situation. Score may include fractions. Retain them. They are important to final score. Convert final score into quality symbol.

and many instructors, as well as many students, operate them with ease. All of them require special handling as well as such special materials as discs, tapes, films or scripts in order to be functional. Often these materials may be obtained through school libraries and, in many cities, through public libraries as well. Almost all state departments of health publish film lists. In addition, the ANA-NLN Film Service of the American Nurses' Association and the National League for Nursing (10 Columbus Circle, New York, N.Y. 10019), publishes a catalogue entitled *Films and Other Visual Resources—for Nursing and Health*. Such professional magazines as *Nursing Outlook* also carry sections on teaching aids to advise readers where and how special films may be obtained on a rental basis.

In recent years, increasingly widespread use is being made of video tapes that may be telecast to schools of nursing over local television stations or closed circuit television. One organization that has been providing this kind of teaching aid is Chicago Video Nursing which is administered by the Evanston (Illinois) Hospital. Its courses consist of series of ten or more lessons, each approximately 45 minutes in length. They are intended to be used "in a working relationship with subjects discussed by the classroom instructor," and a *Students' Study Guide* and *Instructors' Manual* is furnished for each course.

Textbooks probably have the greatest importance and value of all teaching and learning aids. They deal with almost all clinical subjects and there may be several books that deal with the same clinical subject. Nursing school libraries are apt to have a wide selection of them on their shelves. Textbooks are extensively advertised in the *American Journal of Nursing* and *Nursing Outlook* which also carry reviews of new books in each issue. Instructors depend on textbooks and regard them as indispensable sources of reference. Some instructors consider certain textbooks more useful than others and may recommend them to their students for purchase. Other instructors may encourage students to examine and try to use different books dealing with the same subject and then purchase the one (or ones) that seem to meet their needs.

REALITIES

Magazines dealing with almost every clinical subject are published practically every month; some, every week. Like books, they are invaluable current sources of reference and constitute a major part of every medical and nursing library's acquisitions.

Manikins and models are important, too, as teaching and learning aids. Nursing schools all have at least one human skeleton in a closet, and both instructors and students have subjected "Mrs. Chase" to bed baths and treatments of all kinds since time immemorial.

Models of anatomical parts of the body may be purchased from commercial companies who generally advertise them in medical and nursing journals and display them at conventions of professional nursing and medical organizations. Instructors occasionally create models for their own use or inspire their students to make them.

Pamphlets, charts, pictorial folders and mimeographed materials are other aids to teaching and learning. They deal with almost every imaginable clinical subject. Many are available, free of charge or for a minimal fee, from federal, state and local government health agencies; voluntary national, state and local organizations; and through manufacturers of drug and patient care products, as well as through commercial companies dealing in medical, nursing and health supplies.

Lists of publications that are available through the Federal Government may be obtained from the Superintendent of Documents, U.S. Government Printing Office, Washington, D.C. 20402. Publication lists are also available from the American Nurses' Association and from the National League for Nursing, both located at 10 Columbus Circle, New York, N.Y. 10019. Addresses of state nursing organizations and state health departments that also provide visual and other teaching materials, are listed in the Official Directories published in the March and October issues of *Nursing Outlook,* and in the January and August issues of the *American Journal of Nursing* (10 Columbus Circle, New York, N.Y. 10019).

Instructors who are endowed with ability to sketch have a built-in teaching and learning aid. Diagrams they may draw on the blackboard in class to illustrate a process or relationship are meaningful to students and often clarify a concept in a way that words alone cannot do.

All these aids—supplies, furnishings, films and publications—are expedients that the instructor may use to facilitate her students' learning and, as such, are invaluable aspects of the realities in the teaching situation.

V

Summary

Clinical teaching in nursing is envisioned as a goal-directed activity, designed to bring about change in the student's status quo. It is a practice discipline. This means that it is guided by a prescriptive theory that specifies the concepts which influence the instructor's action and enable her to obtain the results she desires through what she does. The instructor is recognized as the formulator of the theory that underlies her teaching as well as the implementor of the concepts it comprehends. Thus, when an explicit prescriptive theory guides her teaching, she gains stability and focus for her action and has the basis for making it ever more meaningful for her students. In presenting clinical teaching in the context of a prescriptive theory, its many facets are laid bare. The instructor's responsibilities are brought into sharp focus, the effect of extraneous forces on her teaching is given recognition, and the many direct and indirect ways by which she influences students and supports their learning efforts are suggested and described.

Three components constitute a prescriptive theory in a clinical teaching context: 1) the instructor's central purpose in teaching; 2) her prescription for fulfilling it; and 3) the realities in clinical teaching—those all-encompassing factors that are present in every situation and that influence the instructor's action and its value to her students.

The central purpose in clinical teaching, founded on the philosophy permeating the tenor of this book, is: to motivate the student and/or facilitate her efforts to overcome the obstacles that now—or may later—interfere with her ability to gain the knowledge, skills and insights she needs in order to function capably, as a nurse, within the realities of the situation of which she is, or may become, a part. This statement of purpose is presented with the thought that clinical instructors may find it of interest as they consider their own beliefs and values and formulate statements of their purposes. Central purpose may be regarded as the instructor's basic reason for engaging in clinical teaching. It specifies her concept of her commitments and suggests the way she thinks she best may go about attaining the results she desires. This central purpose is teamed with her central purpose in nursing, but in a dominant way. It is founded on her philosophy—her beliefs and values—and thus is both a personal and a functional concept. It is also subject to refinements that she makes as new insights sharpen her perspective.

Prescription specifies the kind of action that the instructor believes will most likely lead to fulfillment of her central purpose. Three types of action—mutually understood and agreed-upon, student-directed and instructor-directed—have been identified and their geneses described and diagrammed. The effect each may have on the student has also been suggested, with the conclusion that, although the instructor may, on occasion, resort to student-directed or instructor-directed actions, mutually understood and agreed-upon action is most apt to engender in the student a receptive attitude toward her teaching.

The realities represent all the factors that are at play in the development and implementation of a clinical teaching program. They influence every action the instructor takes and affect her ability to obtain the kind of results she desires from what she does. They are recognized as essentially five in number and each has been described according to its characteristics, its relevance to clinical teaching and its potential significance to the instructor. The five are: the agent, who is identified as the clinical instructor; the recipient, who is the student; the framework, which represents the complex of tangible and intangible factors that may constrain or liberate the instructor in her action; the goal, which is the educational benefit that the instructor desires her students to derive from the particular activities she plans or initiates in their behalf; and the means, which are the expedients through which the instructor facilitates her students' learning.

In conclusion, a prescriptive theory, when respected in all its aspects, lends dignity and stature to any practice discipline. Thus, the clinical instructor who develops and makes explicit the prescriptive theory that underlies her teaching adds a valuable dimension to her specialty and provides herself with a resource that has potential for both guiding and improving her practice.

References

Argyris, Chris. Some Consequences of Separating Thought from Action. *Ventures, Magazine of the Yale Graduate School* VIII:1, Spring 1968, p. 66.
Brown, Margaret. How Much Do Tests and Grades Motivate Learning? *Nurs. Outlook* 16:10, October 1968, p. 60.
Conant, Lucy H. Closing the Practice-Theory Gap. *Nurs. Outlook* 15:11, November 1967, p. 37.
deTornyay, Rheba and Searight, Mary W. Micro-Teaching in Preparing Faculty. *Nurs. Outlook* 16:3, March 1968, p. 34.
Dickoff, James and James, Patrica A. Power. *Amer. J. Nursing* 68:10, October 1968, p. 2128.
_____. A Theory of Theories: A Position Paper. In Symposium on Theory Development in Nursing. *Nurs. Research* 17:3, May-June 1968, p. 197.
Dickoff, James, James, Patricia A., and Wiedenbach, Ernestine. Theory in a Practice Discipline: Part I. Practice Oriented Theory. *Nurs. Research* 17:5, September-October 1968, p. 415.
_____ Part II. Practice Oriented Research. *Nurs. Research* 17:6, November-December 1968, p. 545.
Geitgey, Doris. Some Thoughts on Team Teaching in Nursing Schools. *Nurs. Outlook* 15:10, October 1967, p. 66.
Ginott, Haim G. *Between Parent and Child.* New York: The Macmillan Company, 1965.
Greenwood, Ernest. The Practice of Science and the Science of Practice. In *The Planning of Change,* edited by Warren G. Bennis et al. New York: Rinehart and Winston, 1961.
Hayter, Jean. Guidelines for Selecting Learning Experiences. *Nurs. Outlook* 15:12, December 1967, p. 63.
Layton, Sister Mary Michele. How Instructors' Attitudes Affect Students. *Nurs. Outlook* 17:1, January 1969, p. 27.
Lenahan, Mildred. Looking for Teaching Aids? *Nurs. Outlook* 16:10, October 1968, p. 48.
McBride, Mary Angela B. Facilitating a Masters Program's Clinical Experience. *Nurs. Outlook* 16:11, November 1968, p. 42.
Palmer, Mary Ellen. Self-Evaluation of Clinical Performance. *Nurs. Outlook* 15:11, November 1967, p. 63.

Quint, Jeanne C. Hidden Hazards for Nurse Teachers. *Nurs. Outlook* 15:4, April 1967, p. 34.
Searight, Mary W. A Planning Laboratory. *Nurs. Outlook* 15:12, December 1967, p. 58.
Smith, Dorothy. *Perspectives in Clinical Teaching*. New York: Springer Publishing Company, 1968.
Smith, Dorothy M. A Clinical Nursing Tool. *Amer. J. Nursing* 68:11, November 1968, p. 2384.
Stewart, Ruth F., and Graham, Josephine L. Evaluation Tools in Public Health Nursing Education. *Nurs. Outlook* 16:3, March 1968, p. 50.
Wiedenbach, Ernestine. *Family-Centered Maternity Nursing*, 2nd Edition. New York: G. P. Putnam's Sons, 1967.
_____. *Clinical Nursing—A Helping Art*. New York: Springer Publishing Company, 1964.

Index

A

Ability, 57, 58
Action
　conditioned, 12, 13, 14
　genesis of, 15 (diagram)
　impulsive, 12, 13, 14
　instructor (practitioner) and, 3, 4 (diagram), 8, 14, 16, 17 (diagram), 25 (diagram), 158
　mutually understood and agreed-upon, 3, 4 (diagram), 16, 17 (diagram), 25 (diagram), 158
　reflex, 12, 14
　student (recipient) and, 3, 4 (diagram), 16, 17 (diagram), 25 (diagram), 158
Agent, 4, 19, 21, 24, 158
Analysis, 121
Anxiety, 67, 74, 78, 80, 81
Argyris, Chris, 70
Assignments, 102, 103, 121, 122, *see also* Student
Assumption
　action and, 11, 12, 13
　commitment and, 21, 22
　instructor and, 14, 15, 24, 52, 70, 71
　student and, 72, 77, 81
Attitude, 62, 75, 81, 96, 100
Attributes, 45–49, 46 (sample set), 51, 57, 60

B

Behavior, 75, 100, 101, 130, 132

C

Brake (strategy), 12, 14, 15 (in diagram)

Charting, 116
Classes
　clinical experience and, 30, 43, 107
　conferences and, 103, 104
　instructor and, 31, 103, 105
　student and, 43, 96, 106
Clinical experience, 31, 35, 36, 78, 106
Commitment, 4, 17, 21, 22, 158
Communication, 32, 33
Competence
　desirable student attributes and, 46
　objectives and, 26
　practice and, 32, 63
　student and, 11, 29, 70, 71, 107
　tests and, 143
Concepts, 9, 80, 81, 105, 106
Conferences
　briefing, 114
　group, 36
　individual, 36, 73, 116
　post-experience, 43, 107, 120, 121
　pre-experience, 43, 96, 107
　preparatory, 107
　reconstructions and, 121
Course of study, 28, 29, 31, 62
Critique, 113

D

Deliberateness, 46

163

INDEX

Demonstrations, 109, 110
Discipline, *see* Practice
Discussion, 104–106, 135–137

E

Energy, 57, 59, 71
Evaluation, 44, 103, 142
Examinations, *see* Tests

F

Facilities-for-functioning, 75, 77
Films, 154
Framework
  clinical teaching and, 83
  defined, 4
  goal and, 95, 97
  instructor and, 24, 83, 94, 97
  realities and, 19, 137, 158
  students and, 83, 87, 90, 94, 101

G

Goal
  articulation of, 95
  attainment of, 96, 101, 118, 143, 147
    in-application, 96, 97, 99, 101, 118, 137
    in-execution, 96, 99, 101, 137
    in-intent, 96, 101, 137
  prescriptive theory and, 2, 95, 158
  purpose and, 2, 95
  realities and, 19, 95, 96, 99, 158
  tests and, 143, 145
Grades, 44, 47, 48, 80, 151

H

Head nurse, 40, 42, 53, 108, 110

I

Inconsistencies, 75, 130, 132
Informative material, 37
Instructor
  agent and, 21, 24, 158
  assumptions and, 15, 24, 52, 70, 71
  attributes of, 57, 60
  classes and, 31, 103, 105
  clinical practice and, 34, 60, 61, 62, 63
  commitment and, 21, 22
  conflict of interest and, 6
  framework and, 24, 83, 94, 97
  goal and, 9, 25, 26, 95, 96, 101, 107
  objectives and, 21, 25, 26
  patient and, 6, 8, 60, 115
  prescriptive theory and, 118, 157, 159
  purpose and, 6, 8, 10, 15, 16, 17, 57, 157
  qualifications of, 22
  realities and, 18, 19, 20, 55, 60, 99, 158
  research and, 61, 64
  role of, 23
  student and, 6, 11, 14, 54, 67, 70, 74, 117
  study and, 61, 62
  summary of thinking and, 73, 138–142
  writing and, 60, 64, 65

J

Judgment, 8, 33, 60, 71, 72, 119

K

Knowledge, 29, 71, 143

L

Laboratory ("nursing"), 19
Learning, 1, 34, 48, 49, 81
Lecture, 104

M

Mannikins, 155
Means
  clinical experience and, 106
  defined, 4
  instructor and, 25, 102
  learning aids as, 102, 103, 152, 159
  realities and, 19
Models, 155

INDEX

Motivation, 58, 71, 75

N

Need for help, 31, 58, 125, 130, 132
Nursing, 2, 19, 60, 62
Nursing staff
  clinical teaching and, 52, 53
  instructor and, 35, 52, 53, 63
  planning and, 29, 37, 38

O

Objectives, 21, 25, 26, 31
Observation, 32, 33, 117

P

Patient
  instructor and, 6, 8, 60, 115
  need for help and, 40, 115
  student and, 32, 33, 40, 41, 77, 81, 115, 117
Perception
  assumption and, 12, 14, 15, 24
  conditioned action and, 12, 13
  student and, 78, 132
Philosophy, 4, 15, 23, 157, 158
Planning, Plans
  clinical experience and, 29, 32, 36, 38, 39
  clinical teaching and, 28, 54, 55
  implementation of, 55–60
Practice
  discipline, 2, 3, 4, 11, 103, 157, 159
  improvement of, 60, 64, 65, 159
  instructor and, 60, 61, 62, 63
  realities and, 5
  rehearsal for, 36, 38, 110–114
  tutorial, 107, 115
Practitioner, 2, 4, 95
Prescription
  clinical teaching and, 11, 14
  described, 3, 11, 17
  practice discipline and, 3, 4
  prescriptive theory and, 2, 5
  purpose and, 3, 17, 21, 103, 158
Prescriptive theory
  clinical teaching and, 103, 157
  components of, 2, 5, 157
  discussion and, 136

  practice discipline and, 2, 157, 159
Procedures, 33, 117
Projects, 135, 138
Publication lists, 155
Purpose
  ability and, 58
  action and, 11, 15, 16
  assumptions and, 18, 21, 59
  clinical teaching and, 6, 8, 9, 11, 21, 59, 157
  goal and, 2, 95
  instructor and, 6, 8, 10, 15, 16, 17, 57, 157
  nursing and, 6, 8, 58, 158
  objectives and, 26
  philosophy and, 157, 158
  prescription and, 3, 17, 21, 103, 158
  prescriptive theory and, 2, 5, 103, 136, 157
  student and, 75, 81

R

Realities
  action and, 11, 15
  assumptions and, 21, 22
  clinical teaching and, 18, 19, 20, 158
  described, 4, 18
  instructor and, 18, 19, 20, 55, 60, 99, 158
  judgment and, 33
  practice discipline and, 2, 103
  prescriptive theory and, 2, 5, 137, 157
  professional practice and, 5
  reconstructions and, 124
  rehearsal for practice and, 110
  student experience and, 31
Recipient, 4, 19, 24, 66, 137, 158
Reconstructions, 123–135
Rehearsal for practice, 36–38, 110–114
Reporting, 116
Research, 61, 64
Resourcefulness, 46
Responsibleness, 46
Rounds, 108, 109

S

Score, 48, 50 (sample form), 51 (graphic record), 52, 152, 153 (sample form)
Seminar, 106
Sensations, 12, 15 (in diagram)
Student
  anxiety and, 67, 74, 78, 80, 81
  assignments and, 66, 74, 121
  assumptions and, 72, 77, 81
  attributes and, 45, 46, 47, 48, 49, 51
  behavior and, 75, 100, 101
  clinical experience and, 31, 35, 36, 78, 106
  competence and, 11, 29, 70, 71, 107
  concepts and, 80, 81, 105
  conferences and, 36, 43, 96, 116, 120
  continuity of service and, 41
  discussion and, 105, 106, 135, 136, 137
  framework and, 83, 87, 90, 94, 101
  grades and, 47, 80
  help and, 72, 74, 115, 117
  instructor and, 72, 74, 75, 80, 81, 116, 117
  judgment and, 71, 72
  nursing staff and, 52, 53
  patient and, 32, 33, 40, 41, 77, 81, 115, 117
  preparation and, 35, 36, 78
  prescriptive theory and, 118, 120

purpose and, 75, 81
receptivity and, 100, 101
recipient as, 24, 66
rehearsal for practice and, 36, 110–114
rotation and, 39
thinking and, 34, 105
Study, 61, 62, *see also* Course of Study
Summaries of thinking, 67–70, 82, 138–142
Symbols, 44, 47, 48, 49

T

Teaching aids, 103, 152
Theory, 2, 3, 64, *see also* Prescriptive Theory
Tests, 103, 142–152
Text books, 154
Time schedules, 29, 39–44, 54
Tours, 37, 107

U

Understanding, 46, 57, 59, 71, 75

V

Values, 2, 58, 59, 158
Video-tapes, 154

W

Writing, 60, 64, 65